Vaccines in Society

Tom Douglass · Alistair Anderson

Vaccines in Society

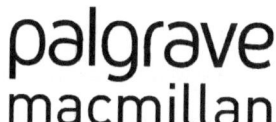

Tom Douglass
University of Birmingham
Birmingham, UK

Alistair Anderson
University of Nottingham
Nottingham, UK

ISBN 978-3-031-61268-8   ISBN 978-3-031-61269-5   (eBook)
https://doi.org/10.1007/978-3-031-61269-5

Cover illustration: © John Rawsterne/patternhead.com

This Palgrave Macmillan imprint is published by the registered company Springer Nature Switzerland AG
The registered company address is: Gewerbestrasse 11, 6330 Cham, Switzerland

If disposing of this product, please recycle the paper.

Acknowledgements

Tom Douglass: This book was written during a period of great happiness and calm in my life for which my partner, Abbie, is in no small part responsible. I am professionally grateful to Professor Michael Calnan. His academic guidance over nearly a decade has been invaluable as have been the countless opportunities he has generated for me. (Alistair and I are additionally thankful for his constructive comments on this book.) I am also indebted to Professor Jon Glasby and the 'Achieving Closure' team at the University of Birmingham who offered me the chance to continue my career at a world-class institution. Finally, the years of love, encouragement and support provided by my parents, Janet and Mike, underpin any achievement.

Alistair Anderson: Between starting and finishing this book, I have made the significant professional change of moving out of academia and into the big wide professional world beyond. My wife, Shannon, has been an ever-present steady support for which I am eternally grateful as I grapple with new challenges, existential questions and my continuing academic commitments in my evenings and weekends. I would be in no position to have helped write this book or pursue the intellectually invigorating career I have enjoyed so far without the support and encouragement of my parents, Susan and Gerard, who must share credit (or possibly blame!) for my achievements along the way.

CONTRIBUTIONS

Tom Douglass and Alistair Anderson are joint first authors. Both contributed equally to the development of the ideas and writing that comprise this book.

CONTENTS

Contents

About the Authors

Tom Douglass is a research fellow at the University of Birmingham. He is a sociologist by background and has research interests within health and social care. He has worked on a broad range of qualitative and mixed-methods research projects concerned with vaccine hesitancy, patient complaints and care home closures.

Alistair Anderson is a geographer with research interests in health behaviours and veterinary medicine. As a mixed-methods social researcher, he has worked on projects concerning antibiotic stewardship, vaccine hesitancy and the experience of work in the veterinary profession.

CHAPTER 1

Vaccines as Social and Political Phenomena?

Abstract The study of vaccine hesitancy has dominated the social analysis of vaccines and the relationship between society and vaccines. Unfortunately, less sustained analytical attention has been given to many of the other social and political dimensions and consequences of vaccines. In this chapter, we set out the benefits of a wider focus within the social scientific analysis of vaccines. We argue that by looking across the composition and operation of what Kirkland has called the immunisation social order, we can reveal the social and political nature of vaccines themselves and the societal consequences or impacts that become visible during or after their development and use.

Keywords Immunisation Social Order · Pharmaceutical Life Course · Vaccine Hesitancy · Vaccine Politics · Social Science

1.1 Introduction

Vaccines are one of public health's foremost tools in the prevention and mitigation of infectious diseases. Vaccines have reduced the incidence and harm of a broad range of deadly and debilitating diseases and their effective deployment is credited with the eradication of smallpox and rinderpest. Recently, vaccines and vaccination were thrust into the centre

T. Douglass and A. Anderson, *Vaccines in Society*, https://doi.org/10.1007/978-3-031-61269-5_1

of public consciousness as part of the policy response to the COVID-19 pandemic (Calnan & Douglass, 2022). COVID-19 vaccines were positioned from the very early stages of the pandemic—and even when COVID-19 vaccines were only in the initial stages of their development—as the way to end restrictions on social and economic life and the best way in the medium term to protect the vulnerable. Readers of this book may themselves have hoped for the expedited development of a COVID-19 vaccine during the long months of lockdown in 2020 and 2021 to return life to 'normal'.

The World Health Organisation recommends that 95% of children in a nation-state are inoculated against vaccine-preventable diseases. Recent data from 2021 to 2022 suggest, however, that none of the routine childhood vaccinations offered in the UK, for example, met this target (Nuffield Trust, 2023). Why is this? Vaccines provoke negative reactions, controversy, hesitancy and even rejection and condemnation from some. One narrative to explain the refusal of vaccine-critical people is that they lack an educated understanding of the benefit, efficacy and safety of vaccination. Analysis by scholars of science and technology studies (STS) and science communication demonstrates, however, that this simplistic deficit narrative insufficiently explains the situation (see, for example, Caudill, 2023, pp. 62–68). Hesitancy and vaccine-critical perceptions and responses are shaped by rather more complex assemblages of social processes and interactions. Indeed, in a book-length examination of this issue, Goldenberg (2021) has powerfully argued that vaccine hesitancy is the result of a crisis of trust, rather than public ignorance or a wider assault on scientific truth.

The study of vaccine hesitancy has dominated the social analysis of vaccines and the relationship between society and vaccines. In addition to academic social scientific concerns about trust and the epistemic basis of science communication, this focus undoubtedly stems from the recognition by governments, health authorities and other funders of research of the harm (public health and economic in nature) caused by low levels of vaccine coverage and the requirement for public buy-in for vaccination programmes to work effectively. With the aim of improving or maintaining high levels of vaccination coverage in the population, considerable social scientific attention has been given to conceptualising and empirically analysing the nature and causes of vaccine hesitancy and vaccine refusal. There is now a large body of theoretical and empirical research examining the social forces that shape decision-making about vaccines by parents and the public. Sitting alongside Goldenberg (2021), other books on the topic, such as Reich (2016), offer considered analysis of how parents see vaccine refusal, the dimensions and dynamics of their vaccine hopes and fears and their promotion of health and 'natural immunity' instead of vaccination. Larson (2020), meanwhile, focuses on the cultural conditions that perpetuate vaccine rumour and misinformation. Larson argues that "debunking rumours, one rumour at a time, will not fix the questioning and convictions. It is too late for that. What is needed is a more fundamental change around the fertile ground which is fuelling the concerns, rumours, and heated debates" (Larson, 2020, p. xxviii). Together these examples—and this is by no means an exhaustive list— illustrate the complexity of vaccine hesitancy and the concern with which it is treated as a challenge to vaccine uptake.

From the very first vaccine to protect against smallpox through to the recent COVID-19 vaccines, the development and use of vaccines have attracted public dispute and debate. Many of the views that exist today about vaccines have persisted since vaccination's inception. At different times, in different combinations and in relation to specific vaccines and vaccination programmes, people have believed that "vaccines are ineffective or cause diseases; vaccines are used to make profit; vaccines contain dangerous substances; harms caused by vaccines are hidden by the authorities; vaccination mandates violate civil rights; natural immunity is better than immunity induced by vaccines or natural approaches to health and alternative products (e.g., homeopathy, vitamins) are superior to vaccines to prevent diseases" (Dubé et al., 2015, p. 106). Vaccines therefore intertwine with a range of health, economic, governmental and social justice concerns in the public conscious.

The vaccine hesitancy evidence base reveals that safety concerns alongside (dis)trust in vaccines, health authorities, the pharmaceutical industry and the medical profession are central components in parental and public attitudes towards vaccines (Attwell et al., 2017; Goldenberg, 2021; Hobson-West, 2007; Yaqub et al., 2014). Moreover, vaccination is tensely positioned between notions of individual rights and social responsibilities—the individual's right to choose and the responsibility to protect the health of others within the collective (Larson, 2020, p. 62) and between persuasion and compulsion (Colgrove, 2006). A growing emphasis on choice and individual responsibility—in both medicine specifically and in society more generally under the conditions of neoliberalism—sits uneasily alongside the community focus of vaccination as do compulsory approaches to vaccination adopted by health authorities. Approaches and attitudes towards risk, past vaccination and wider medical experiences and historical factors can also influence parental and public understandings and vaccine uptake (see Calnan & Douglass, 2020 for further detail).

Unfortunately, however, less sustained analytical attention has been given to the broader social and political dimensions and consequences of vaccines; a wider lens is needed.

1.2   A Conceptual Approach

In modern capitalist societies, there exists what we can think of as an 'immunisation social order' (see Kirkland, 2016). Kirkland (2016) centres the socio-legal dimensions of the immunisation social order and its preservation in her empirical analysis—in particular, the work of the 'vaccine court' that adjudicates on vaccine injury in the USA context (a topic we engage with in Chapter 2). Kirkland shows us that the immunisation social order reveals a broader yet fragile web of institutional, scientific, legal—and importantly—social, and political practices, associated actors, values and relationships that produce and protect high levels of vaccination coverage (ibid.). In her own words, Kirkland is concerned with "the role of law in channelling social movement conflict and resolving the challenges that vaccine injuries pose to [the] immunisation social order" (2016, p. 3).

Though Kirkland's concept of the immunisation social order has emerged from socio-legal studies (with an associated empirical interest in the uniquely positioned 'vaccine court' in the USA), we argue that this concept has broader social scientific potential. We suggest that it is an important concept as it directs analytical attention beyond the primacy of vaccine hesitancy as the grounds for social scientific engagement to the broader network of factors that shape how societies maintain high levels of vaccination coverage as well as the full breadth of social forces that threaten vaccination or that may prevent high levels of vaccination coverage. We argue that by looking across the immunisation social order in this way and including dimensions that have thus far been neglected or under-analysed, we can simultaneously reveal the broad social and political nature of vaccines themselves and the societal consequences or impacts that become visible during or after their development and use. Though some of the evidence we draw on is relevant only to the functioning of or challenges to the immunisation social order within a specific country, there are also international implications revealed by the analysis.

The focus in social research on the reasons why people hold vaccine-critical views and/or may not wish to vaccinate themselves or their children is of course important but is limited in that it is only able to improve understandings of one dimension and set of challenges to the immunisation social order. What the body of research concerned with vaccine hesitancy has often failed to systematically attend to is that values, relations, processes and politics are embedded at every stage of the 'pharmaceutical life course' of a vaccine (Casper & Carpenter, 2008), including their development, production, licensing, marketing, mediatisation, allocation and use. In this regard, we are also influenced by Casper and Carpenter (2008) who encourage analysis of how "at every stage of their life courses... pharmaceuticals may influence politics and social relations, which in turn may (re)shape the technology itself. [Indeed, pharmaceutical technologies] can instigate political struggles, and potentially social change, over time" (Carpenter & Casper, 2009, p. 794). Built into this approach is recognition that social and political forces "shape the ways [pharmaceutical technologies] are produced, used, and so forth; but [that these technologies] may also instigate political struggles, and, potentially, social change, over their life courses, as well as embodying extant conflicts" (Casper & Carpenter, 2008, p. 887).

Our aim in this book is to assemble and reframe evidence from medical sociology, science and technology studies, public health, health geography and the medical humanities relating to the social and political nature of vaccines and discuss the consequences for society's continued engagement with vaccines. Our approach is to look at the embeddedness and influence of social and political values and relations relating to a broad range of significant and some relatively neglected elements of the immunisation social order from across the breadth of the life course of vaccines. To this end, we critically discuss vaccine development and regulation, the mediatisation of vaccines, vaccine inequalities and non-human animals' relationship to the technology of vaccines.

This comprehensive analysis of the social and political nature and impacts of vaccines—extracting a range of insights from literatures never gathered in this manner before—is significant. It helps us answer questions related to the composition, functioning, maintenance of and challenges to or within the immunisation social order; for example, how social values shape the development and use of specific vaccines and in turn how culture and society may be reshaped by new vaccines, the dynamics of power and the interests served in vaccination policy, the role of various forms of media in co-producing the nature and understandings of vaccines, the consequences of inequalities in access to and uptake of vaccines and the relationships between human and non-human actors in the development and use of vaccines. Furthermore, we ultimately argue that appropriately situating the issue of vaccine hesitancy in this broader social and political analysis can ultimately deepen our understanding of this phenomenon and how it is shaped by values, processes and relationships situated in or connected to other elements of the immunisation social order.

The COVID-19 pandemic simultaneously demonstrated the value of vaccination as a public health intervention while illuminating and reconfiguring the social and political dimensions of vaccines—notably, for example, how vaccine development is funded, how vaccine safety is ensured, as well as the inequalities in access to vaccines in an initial context of limited supply (Calnan & Douglass, 2022). As the emergency phase of the COVID-19 pandemic recedes and new evidence about the role of vaccines in society becomes available, we argue that it is now prudent to (re)examine evidence relating to the nature of the social and political values, interests and relations embedded in and reshaped by the development, regulation, allocation and use of vaccines.

1.3   STRUCTURE OF THE BOOK

Across the following chapters, we analyse the social and political factors shaping the emergence, nature and functioning of the immunisation social order while also revealing its tensions, restrictions and challenges. The next chapter examines the history of vaccines and is designed to historically contextualise discussions later in the book. Via Edward Jenner and smallpox vaccination and concluding in the early neoliberal era, it is the story of the social and political dimensions central to the history of vaccines and vaccine science over the last two centuries.

Chapter 3 explores examples of how subjective values and social relations influence and (re)shape the interconnected processes of development and regulation. First, the chapter begins with an overview of the central actors and processes in the development and regulatory assessment of vaccines. Following this we turn to analyse vaccines as political entities discussing how gendered and heteronormative values were embedded in and were then influenced by the development and subsequent public response to the first human papillomavirus (HPV) vaccine. The chapter similarly discusses the political nature of vaccines in relation to national security. Next, the chapter looks at the case of RotaShield, the first vaccine developed to prevent rotavirus. This case highlights the importance of subjective values in regulatory assessment and the ultimate withdrawal of the RotaShield vaccine from the market. Finally, the chapter explores the development of COVID-19 vaccines analysing the relationships between powerful actors and showing how the interests of these powerful groups were reflected in the approaches to development and regulatory assessment.

Chapter 4 examines the role of mass and social media in public discourse around vaccines and vaccination. The chapter begins by outlining why mass media play an important role in the public consciousness regarding vaccines and vaccination, using examples from the recent history of vaccines to illustrate the role of journalists in the co-production of how we know and understand vaccines. Following this the role of social media and the growing field of social media analytics for the maintenance of high levels of vaccination coverage is examined, with attention given to the new possibilities that social media provides for social research and some of the challenges and limitations that are yet to be overcome in the field.

Being situated within society means being positioned within a broad coalition of social, political and economic power relations that lend generous advantage to certain groups while radically disadvantaging others. In Chapter 5, we examine how these advantages and disadvantages intersect with the public health imperative of maximal vaccine uptake. The chapter begins by exploring the impact of vaccination on social inequalities, highlighting that though the primary goal of vaccination is to reduce the incidence of mortality and morbidity from disease, vaccination can also reduce social inequalities. The chapter then turns to examine the inequalities that shape access to vaccination and vaccination uptake. This is analysed in two ways, firstly looking at international inequalities in vaccine access through the recent example of the COVID-19 pandemic, and secondly by considering sub-national social inequalities in vaccine access and uptake.

In Chapter 6, we explore a dimension of vaccination that has received disparate and sporadic attention from the social sciences—the interconnectedness of non-human animals with the technology of vaccination.

The chapter opens by outlining the rationale for social scientists' engagement with animals before then considering the role of animals in vaccine development, and the use of vaccines to mitigate the ever-growing threat of epizootics. This examination is framed using the concept of 'One Health'. We then discuss how the use of vaccines in relation to non-human animals is tied to an important medical history: the professionalisation of veterinary medicine. Expertise in the treatment of animal diseases and the use of vaccines to address key public health concerns have been key tools used historically by the veterinary profession to demarcate their professional territory from, for example, medical doctors and farriers.

References

Attwell, K., Leask, J., Meyer, S. B., Rokkas, P., & Ward, P. (2017). Vaccine rejecting parents' engagement with expert systems that inform vaccination programs. *Journal of Bioethical Inquiry, 14*(1), 65–76. https://doi.org/10.1007/s11673-016-9756-7

Calnan, M., & Douglass, T. (2020). Hopes, hesitancy and the risky business of vaccine development. *Health, Risk & Society, 22*(5–6), 291–304. https://doi.org/10.1080/13698575.2020.1846687

Calnan, M., & Douglass, T. (2022). *Power, policy and the pandemic: A sociological analysis of COVID-19 policy in England*. Emerald Publishing Limited.

Carpenter, L. M., & Casper, M. J. (2009). A tale of two technologies: HPV vaccination, male circumcision, and sexual health. *Gender & Society, 23*(6), 790–816. https://doi.org/10.1177/0891243209352490

Casper, M. J., & Carpenter, L. M. (2008). Sex, drugs, and politics: The HPV vaccine for cervical cancer. *Sociology of Health & Illness, 30*(6), 886–899. https://doi.org/10.1111/j.1467-9566.2008.01100.x

Caudill, D. S. (2023). *Expertise in crisis: The ideological contours of public scientific controversies*. Policy Press.

Colgrove, J. (2006). *State of immunity: The politics of vaccination in twentieth century America*. University of California Press.

Dubé, E., Vivion, M., & MacDonald, N. E. (2015). Vaccine hesitancy, vaccine refusal and the anti-vaccine movement: Influence, impact and implications. *Expert Review of Vaccines, 14*(1), 99–117. https://doi.org/10.1586/14760584.2015.964212

Goldenberg, M. J. (2021). *Vaccine hesitancy: Public trust, expertise, and the war on science*. University of Pittsburgh Press.

Hobson-West, P. (2007). 'Trusting blindly can be the biggest risk of all': Organised resistance to childhood vaccination in the UK. *Sociology of Health &*

Illness, 29(2), 198–215. https://doi.org/10.1111/j.1467-9566.2007.005
44.x

Kirkland, A. (2016). *Vaccine court: The law and politics of injury.* NYU Press.

Larson, H. J. (2020). *Stuck: How vaccine rumours start—And why they don't go away.* Oxford University Press.

Nuffield Trust. (2023). *Vaccination coverage for children and mothers.* https://www.nuffieldtrust.org.uk/resource/vaccination-coverage-for-children-and-mothers-1

Reich, J. A. (2016). *Calling the shots.* New York University Press.

Yaqub, O., Castle-Clarke, S., Sevdalis, N., & Chataway, J. (2014). Attitudes to vaccination: A critical review. *Social Science & Medicine, 112*, 1–11. https://doi.org/10.1016/j.socscimed.2014.04.018

CHAPTER 2

The Emerging Immunisation Social Order: A History of Vaccines

Abstract This chapter is a historical account of the social and political dimensions of vaccines and vaccine science over the last two centuries. Beginning with Benjamin Jesty, Edward Jenner and smallpox vaccination and concluding in the early neoliberal era, the chapter provides an overview of the social stories at the centre of the history of vaccinology. We show that the socioeconomic and political conditions of the day have shaped vaccine development and access—that the march of vaccinology has not occurred in a social vacuum—with new vaccines or the need for new vaccines in turn reshaping society. In this regard, this chapter begins the process of highlighting the growth of the immunisation social order which contextualises discussions later in the book. We also consider the history of challenges, restrictions or problems within the immunisation social order. Though vaccination has undoubtedly saved many lives across its history, the path from the first vaccine to the plethora of vaccines in use today has been marked by considerable and frequent controversy. In this regard, we also begin to explore how social and political values and the interests held by social actors have influenced and reshaped vaccine controversy and the nature and functioning of the immunisation social order.

Keywords Social History of Vaccines · Vaccine Development · Vaccine Controversy · Neoliberalism · Edward Jenner

© The Author(s), under exclusive license to Springer Nature Switzerland AG 2024
T. Douglass and A. Anderson, *Vaccines in Society*,
https://doi.org/10.1007/978-3-031-61269-5_2

11

2.1   Introduction

This chapter is a historical account of the social and political dimensions of vaccines and vaccine science over the last two centuries. Beginning with Benjamin Jesty, Edward Jenner and smallpox vaccination and concluding in the early neoliberal era, the chapter provides an overview of the social stories at the centre of the history of vaccinology. We show that the socioeconomic and political conditions of the day have shaped vaccine development and access—that the march of vaccinology has not occurred in a social vacuum—with new vaccines or the need for new vaccines in turn reshaping society. In this regard, this chapter begins the process of highlighting the social and political factors shaping the growth of the immunisation social order which contextualises discussions later in the book. We also consider the history of challenges, restrictions or problems within the immunisation social order. Though vaccination has undoubtedly saved many lives across its history, the path from the first vaccine to the plethora of vaccines in use today has been marked by considerable and frequent controversy. In this regard, we also begin to explore how social and political values and the interests held by social actors have influenced and reshaped vaccine controversy and the nature and functioning of the immunisation social order.

There is a long history of anti-vaccination resistance and parental hesitancy towards vaccines that emerged alongside the very first vaccine to protect people against smallpox; resistance and public concern about vaccines has never been absent for very long. However, this dimension of the history of vaccination has been written about at length by others (see, for example, Dubé et al., 2015; Durbach, 2005; Poland & Jacobson, 2001; Reich, 2016, pp. 23–66).[1] As outlined in the introductory chapter, our focus in this book looks beyond only hesitancy and resistance to examine the broader social and political nature and impacts of vaccines.

---

[1] See also Colgrove (2006) for a rich political historical discussion of the trajectory of vaccination policy in the US and the strategies adopted by health authorities to persuade or compel people to accept vaccination.

2.2 THE ORIGINS OF VACCINATION: VARIOLATION, SMALLPOX, JESTY AND JENNER

For many years (certainly as far back as seventeenth-century China) before vaccination was established as a routine procedure, an earlier process known as variolation was used to fight the deadly disease of smallpox (Leung, 2011). This process involved "a lancet wet with fresh matter taken from a ripe pustule of some person who suffered from smallpox. The material was then subcutaneously introduced on the arms or legs of the nonimmune person" (Riedel, 2005, p. 22) to inoculate against smallpox. Though there are some uncertainties regarding the origins and invention of the procedure of variolation, the first written record was in a 1695 medical book authored by a doctor named Zhang Lu. The technique was said to confer 'Taoist immortality' and to have been first practised in Jiangxi before spreading throughout the country during the life of Zhang Lu (Leung, 2011). Power and privilege are also central to the story. Lady Mary Wortley Montagu encountered the practice of variolation during travel to Turkey with her husband who was a British ambassador. Having survived smallpox Montagu insisted her son be variolated later demonstrating the technique to British surgeons. Subsequently, "experiments on the safety of variolation were performed on six prisoners, and later on orphans, and those proving successful, the Princess of Wales asked to have her daughters variolated. Owing to new popularity and the tightly organised practice of medicine in Europe, variolation became widespread" (Reich, 2016, pp. 23–24).

In 1796, Edward Jenner, a doctor in the English countryside, is commonly understood to have invented a vaccination procedure which, by 1840, led to variolation being outlawed in England due to the greater safety of the vaccination process (Riedel, 2005). The story, as often told, is one of Jenner's scientific experimentations leading him to immunise an eight-year-old boy named James Phipps with pus from the cowpox lesion of milkmaid Sarah Nelmes who had told Jenner one of her cows had recently suffered from cowpox (Stern & Markel, 2005; see also Bailey, 2011; Baxby, 2011). Later, the boy was variolated with smallpox and no disease developed. Following further experimentation, Jenner disseminated his findings and became a celebrated and famous figure, and was also rewarded financially by parliament (Stern & Markel, 2005). Until the 1870s, vaccination solely referred to the procedure to protect people against smallpox (the name was derived from 'variolae vaccinae' which was

Jenner's own Latin translation of smallpox of the cow) before taking on its wider meaning in the nineteenth century when Louis Pasteur proposed at the 7th International Congress of Medicine held in London that the term be broadened to include all protective immunisation procedures (Esparza et al., 2020). Smallpox vaccination in the nineteenth century was not the same process as vaccination today; it was certainly not painless, and neither was it a minor medical procedure (Durbach, 2005, p. 3).

Despite the famous account, and though Jenner is undeniably an important figure in the history of vaccination, Pead (2017a, 2017b) shows that he did not achieve vaccination first. More accurately the history of the smallpox vaccine is one of the socially situated nature of knowledge production; in this regard, the first phase in the development of the immunisation social order reflects relationality and social privilege rather than individual scientific genius. Benjamin Jesty, a farmer in Dorset, was influenced by local folk knowledge that milkmaids who contracted cowpox as a result of their work were not subsequently infected with smallpox (Pead, 2006, 2017a, 2017b), and sought to protect the lives of his family members during an outbreak of smallpox in 1774 by transferring material from the udders of cattle that were known to have cowpox to the arms of his wife and children (Baxby, 2011; Riedel, 2005). Thus, Jesty delivered the first recorded vaccinations 22 years before Jenner.[2] Horton (1995) meanwhile explains that Jenner gained priority in the history of vaccination—and that knowledge of vaccination subsequently spread so widely—was primarily due to his position in society compared to farmer Jesty. Not only was Jenner a fellow of the Royal Society for previous, unrelated work on cuckoos, but he was also connected to the aristocracy and Lord Mayor of London. Jesty was eventually recognised in 1805 with two gold mounted lancets and a document demonstrating his discovery of vaccination—but it is Jenner who built fame and fortune from the invention of vaccination and it is Jenner's name that is still closely associated with vaccination today.[3]

[2] The importance of Jesty has more recently come to public attention—due particularly to the efforts of Patrick Pead (see 2017a, 2017b, 2019; see also BBC News, 2021).

[3] However, we should not dismiss Jenner's contribution. His work certainly helped to confer scientific legitimacy on vaccination; he also worked to widely disseminate knowledge about vaccination and laid the groundwork for the scientific field of vaccinology (Riedel, 2005; Stern & Markel, 2005). Additionally, as Reich (2016, p. 25) notes, "Jenner never sold [the] discovery, spent his own money to create and distribute stock of [vaccine] and

2.3 Beyond Smallpox

Nearly a century after Jenner, the meaning of vaccination was broadened through the work of Louis Pasteur. Though the development of smallpox vaccination was highly important, scientific understanding of the development of immunity had not itself significantly developed (Smith, 2012). Work in the 1870s on chicken cholera, anthrax and later rabies introduced the notion that vaccination could be applied broadly to microbial disease. Pasteur and collaborators showed that pathogens could be attenuated (weakened) so that preventative vaccines based on a reproducible method could be made in a laboratory and ultimately manufactured widely (Bazin, 2011). Importantly, before children Joseph Meister and Jean-Baptise Jupille became the first people to be vaccinated against rabies, rabies vaccination had only been conducted on animals. The introduction of a deadly agent into humans through vaccination caused controversy even though these children had been bitten by rabid animals and were likely to die. After several years with many successful vaccinations and saved lives, the opinions of the public and medical establishment swung in favour of rabies vaccination. The foundation of the Pasteur Institute in 1888 highlighted the triumph of Pasteurian ideas.

Löwy (1994) shows that though the Institute was supposed to be a private organisation drawing funding from a broad range of sources, and that Pasteur had stated his desire to be independent from the French state, the Pasteurians relied heavily on government funding for research. The needs of public health were therefore central to the mission of the Institute. Löwy suggests that these arrangements and ideals possibly hampered the development of more highly profitable arrangements with commercial enterprise. However, though the Institute's official ideology was one of 'disinterested' scientific research, it did rely on sales of vaccines to balance its books. As we will explore later in the chapter, the issues of funding vaccine research and balancing the interests of public health and the profit motive are persistent dilemmas within the immunisation social order.

information, and was known to vaccinate the poor in his town free. At great personal cost, Jenner gave up his lifestyle as a physician and family man to become a 'missionary to vaccination'".

In a foundational text within science and technology studies,[4] Latour (1993) argues that Pasteur's methodological triumph cannot be reduced to individual genius. In Latour's (1993, p. 16) own words:

> If, to explain the "diffusion" of Pasteur's ideas, we had nothing more than the force of Pasteur and his collaborators, those ideas would never have left the walls of the Ecole Normale laboratory and would not even have entered them. An idea, even an idea of genius, even an idea that is to save millions of people, never moves of its own accord. It requires a force to fetch it, seize upon it for its own motives, move it, and often transform it.

The success of scientific and technological innovation is considered here the result of relationships between actors including human and non-human actors, such as microbes, their interactions and power relations within a network. Interconnection of Pasteurian laboratory successes in isolating microbes with the hygienist movement and its various components, including environmental and moralistic dimensions, was central to and reshaped by the diffusion and transformation of Pasteurian ideas. Here we can see Latour's contention that nature and society influence and reshape one another; one unreducible to the other.

Robert Koch's Institute for Infectious Diseases in Berlin was also important in the growing bacterial understanding of disease (in which it was recognised that if bacteriology was to be truly valuable, the causative agent of an infectious disease needed to be isolated) during the final years of the nineteenth century and the early years of the twentieth century. As Blume and Baylac-Paouly (2021, p. 3) state, "Pasteur's and Koch's ideas regarding the mechanism of disease causation, and in particular the influence of environmental factors, differed substantially. So too did the structures of the institutes that they directed, reflecting the different political and administrative traditions of the two countries (which had actually been at war with one another only a decade earlier)". Nevertheless, the work of Koch and collaborators facilitated the isolation of the causative agent of the deadly disease of tuberculosis—which has killed more people than any other pathogen (Luca & Mihaescu, 2013). It was in the years afterwards that scientists at the Pasteur Institute in France were able to develop a vaccine for tuberculosis. Albert Calmette and Camille Guérin

---

[4] This work indirectly begins to set out the central contentions of Latour's actor-network theory.

began research into the tuberculosis vaccine in 1900 at the Pasteur Institute. It took until 1913 before they were prepared to initiate a trial of the vaccine in cattle—which was then interrupted by the First World War. Their research continued during German occupation despite difficulties obtaining research materials. By 1921, the vaccine was ready for testing on humans and by 1924, they were able to report a series of 664 oral vaccinations of infants. The Pasteur Institute began the mass production of the Bacille Bilie Calmette-Guérin (BCG) vaccine. By 1928, 114,000 infants had been vaccinated against tuberculosis without serious issue.

However, public confidence in the BCG vaccine was undermined by the Lubeck disaster in Germany. BCG was supplied by the Pasteur Institute but preparation for administering the vaccine for a local vaccination programme of new-born babies took place in the tuberculosis laboratory in Lubeck, Germany where there was subsequently a disaster (Luca & Mihaescu, 2013). Of 250 vaccinated infants, 73 died of tuberculosis within a year and another 135 had been infected but recovered. After an investigation, it was found that contamination had occurred at the Lubeck Laboratory with two doctors consequently given prison sentences. Calmette and Guérin endured criticism because of the disaster. British scientists also initially questioned the safety and value of the tuberculosis vaccine (the BCG vaccine) and it was not immediately adopted in Britain. There was a further cultural moralistic component to this rejection with people encouraged to take responsibility for their own health and eat a healthy diet (Bryder, 1999). The vaccine was initially thought to disincentivise lifestyle change and promote a false sense of security—even though aspects far beyond individual control, such as housing shortages and undernutrition caused by the First World War had exacerbated the impacts of disease. Despite this, the BCG vaccine is still widely used globally today and prevents many deaths from tuberculosis.

2.4 THE GOLDEN AGE

The Second World War and its aftermath led to an intensification of vaccine research resulting in what some have described as the golden age of vaccine development in the Cold War era (Poland & Jacobson, 2011). In an increasingly polarised world, countries across the East/West divide had different visions for how health systems should be organised. Nevertheless, politicians on both sides of the ideological spectrum thought that demonstrating the ability to control infectious disease—or in other words, the development of an effective immunisation social order—would cast their political system in a positive light. Infectious disease was prospering in cities decimated by war with large numbers of displaced people. In this regard, vaccine success was ideologically desirable, and vaccines were weighted with political significance (Blume & Baylac-Paouly, 2021).

Interestingly, it was through collaboration across the 'ideological divide' that there was success in the fights against polio and smallpox (Manela, 2010). In 1956, the US State Department and Soviet counterparts facilitated connections between American and Soviet virologists to collaborate in the production of an oral polio vaccine—with this vaccine subsequently successfully deployed globally. As Hotez (2017, p. 1) notes

> [w]atched closely by a suspected KGB operative, the Russian virologists visited [Dr Albert] Sabin in his Cincinnati Children's Hospital research laboratory, and this was followed by Sabin's reciprocal visit to Moscow in the same year. Within two years, a shipment of Sabin's polio virus strains arrived in the Soviet Union on dry ice.

In 1958 a delegation from the Soviet Union encouraged the WHO to commit to the eradication of smallpox. The Soviet Union had been able to stop the domestic transmission of smallpox, but costly vaccination had to continue as it was imported by immigrants and travellers (smallpox remained widespread in Asia, Africa and parts of Latin America). At the 1965 meeting of the World Health Assembly (the decision-making body of the WHO), the USA supported the Soviet Union's smallpox eradication proposal for which the Director-General of the WHO subsequently drew up a plan. The USA hoped that involvement in such a humanitarian mission would help to lessen the political damage caused by America's involvement in war (Blume & Baylac-Paouly, 2021). The Soviets established a process to preserve smallpox vaccine in harsh environments (Hotez, 2017) which was crucial for distributing the vaccine globally, while the USA provided funding and skilled labour (Blume & Baylac-Paouly, 2021). In this sense, Cold War vaccine diplomacy and collaboration between the USA and the Soviet Union was highly significant in the eradication of smallpox in 1980 and the further development of the immunisation social order (Manela, 2010).

This period also saw an important methodological breakthrough: the growth of viruses in cell culture that could be used in the production of vaccines (Plotkin & Plotkin, 2011). The first licensed vaccine using cell culture technique was for polio in 1955 developed by Jonas Salk. It additionally led to the development of vaccines against measles (1963), mumps (1967) and rubella (1969) (which we return to below). The development of the polio vaccine was also notable in that it represented the first true controlled clinical trial with the vaccine compared against placebo (and an extremely large one at that involving roughly 1.8 million children). Polio vaccine research was significantly funded by the National Foundation for Infant Paralysis (NFIP) founded in 1938 by President Roosevelt (who had been paralysed by polio) and his former law partner Basil O'Connor. The NFIP instituted the March of the Dimes where people nationwide were encouraged to donate a small amount to collectively fund the fight against polio (Reich, 2016, p. 41). Salk did not patent the vaccine and six pharmaceutical companies were given licences to produce the vaccine (ibid.); Salk also shared the detail of the production process with laboratories abroad (Blume & Baylac-Paouly, 2021). The Salk polio vaccine consequently marked "one of the first significant mergers between public research and for-profit pharmaceutical production" in the development of the immunisation social order (Reich, 2016, p. 43). Given the heavy levels of protection afforded to intellectual property in the present day, acts of public donation such as Salk's are relatively rare. However, despite public concern about equitable distribution of polio, in a political culture of fear of communism the US federal government did not manage vaccine distribution and relatedly the American Medical Association and pharmaceutical industry fiercely opposed a 'socialised' approach to vaccination (Oshinsky, 2005).

In the haste to manufacture the vaccine developed by Salk, cases of paralytic polio were found in vaccine recipients, resulting in five children's deaths, because of a manufacturing incident where incomplete attenuation of polio virus had occurred (importantly, the vaccine was not inherently harmful) (Dubé et al., 2015). As a result, the polio vaccination programme in the USA was halted while manufacturing procedures were assessed, and the source of the problem identified. Additional manufacturing steps and greater safety testing were mandated in the industry following this incident. This event became known as the Cutter Incident—named after Cutter Laboratories, the company at the centre of the controversy who had manufactured all the defective doses of vaccine that harmed people. It represents one of the worst pharmaceutical disasters in history (Offit, 2005). Reflecting the strong positive societal sentiment around vaccination at the time, and likely also the fear of the disease, this incident, however, did not significantly impact acceptance of vaccination. Nevertheless, the lawsuits that were subsequently filed did impact pharmaceutical companies for many years to come as the precedent of liability without fault was born (where companies were liable for the effects of their products even if they were not negligent in terms of design or manufacturing process) (Carapetis, 2006). This ultimately led to new legislation to protect manufacturers and the vaccine supply (we return to this issue in the next section).

A rubella vaccine held the promise of solving two major social problems of the day as the 1960s drew to their end. First, during rubella outbreaks many babies were born with birth defects. Second, women in the US would attend hospital review boards to request an abortion claiming that they had been exposed to rubella during pregnancy—with abortion in this historical and cultural context only available for medical necessity. Judgements by committee members were thus central to decision-making as there was no way to verify exposure to rubella during pregnancy. There were fears at the time that some women falsified claims of exposure to rubella to obtain abortions (Reagan, 2012). However, though promising to solve these problems, the rubella vaccine also introduced a new dilemma. Unlike other vaccines the aim was to protect foetuses rather than the individual that received the vaccination. The ethical question that emerged from the development of this vaccine was whether it was acceptable to expose the individual receiving the vaccination to possible adverse effects for the benefit of future foetuses and the wider community—a tension that still exists more generally in vaccination policy and decision-making today (see Calnan & Douglass, 2020).

2.4.1   The Pertussis Vaccine Controversy

The Great Ormond Street Hospital for Sick Children based in London published a report in 1974 (see Kulenkampff et al., 1974) which suggested a link between serious neurological conditions and the diphtheria-tetanus-pertussis (DTP) combination vaccine (which had been in use in Britain for 20 years at this time). The report led to significant media coverage—and clear indication of the important role played by news media in framing and influencing how vaccines are understood as well as disseminating challenges to or problems within the immunisation social order (we return to this discussion in Chapter 4). This coverage included emotive stories of harm allegedly caused by the vaccine—for example, the story of a man left severely disabled after apparent involvement in pertussis vaccine trials in the 1950s (Baker, 2003). In 1974, the Sunday Times (see ibid.), for example, published an article titled "Boy's brain damaged in vaccine experiment". Over time, news coverage of the legal wrangling associated with the controversy contributed to keep it alive in the public imagination, though television and newspaper reports were not necessarily or totally anti-vaccine in tone. Rather journalists were responding to and framing the controversy and drama while seeking to distil a complicated pharmaceutical safety issue being debated in medical journals into an accessible human-interest story (ibid.). The formation of the Association of Parents of Vaccine Damaged Children—during the dispute—shows that the public were far from a passive force manipulated by the news media. The organisation drew further attention to the purported safety problems of the pertussis vaccine, coordinating legal efforts, keeping media attention on the issue and advocating for compensation. Here we can see how the interests, of and relationships between, social actors influenced and reshaped the scope of a vaccine controversy that needed to be overcome during the development of the immunisation social order.

Baker (2003) shows that the incident led to a considerable fall in immunisation rates against pertussis (also known as whooping cough) falling from 77 to 33% nationwide coverage in Britain (and even lower in some parts of the country). Outbreaks of whooping cough soon followed. Another key social dimension in the controversy was the emergence of a divide in the medical community—with some professionals prominently co-operating with anti-vaccine groups. A general ambivalence towards the vaccine was displayed by general practitioners and visiting nurses (ibid.)—although this seems to have reflected a high cultural tolerance in Britain towards both whooping cough which was viewed as relatively benign.

After years of medical and legal dispute, by the end of the 1980s, the controversy was finally losing momentum and vaccination coverage improved. Important here was a legal ruling in 1988 asserting that the evidence of permanent neurological harm was unconvincing. In 1991, a major report from the Institute of Medicine in the US reviewed all medical literature on the topic. It definitively concluded that there was insufficient evidence for an association between pertussis vaccination and permanent neurological damage.

However, the controversy had already spread to other countries in the 1980s. In the USA, an Emmy-award winning documentary entitled

'DPT: Vaccine Roulette' associating the pertussis vaccine with neurological problems was produced while angry and concerned parents formed vaccine-critical organisations and lawsuits against manufacturers were instigated (Dubé et al., 2015). The increased litigation harmed the willingness of manufacturers to produce vaccines and thus threatened the supply of vaccines (an issue we return to below). This represented a significant challenge to the emerging immunisation social order. The controversy led to the creation of the National Childhood Vaccine Injury Compensation Programme in the USA (see Kirkland, 2016) and the Vaccine Adverse Event Report System (VAERS) (see Chapter 3) where adverse effects of vaccines could be reported by health professionals and parents (Dubé et al., 2015).

2.5   Developing Vaccines in the Neoliberal Era

Despite earlier successes, by the 1970s and 1980s, vaccine development was beginning to prove difficult and commercial viability was limited particularly in comparison with the development of new therapeutic drugs. It also became clear that there were heightened risks associated with vaccine development and rigorous testing was necessary. Fears among vaccine manufacturers emerged relating to severe liability claims. A small number of people are harmed by vaccination (e.g. by an allergic reaction), but the pharmaceutical industry argued that even a small number of compensation claims in civil court could be ruinous for companies—and thus drive up prices or harm even the supply of established vaccines (Blume, 2017: see 149–151).

Reflecting the withdrawal of many pharmaceutical companies from vaccine development at this time, and fears that the supply of vaccines might be badly disrupted, several changes subsequently occurred that shape vaccine development and production today and thus the nature and composition of the immunisation social order. Governments developed statutory provisions to compensate individuals harmed by vaccines (litigation was of particular concern in the USA) (Blume, 2017). These programmes were designed to protect and limit the liability of vaccine manufacturers in the event of serious adverse effects. This is known as the Vaccine Damage Payment (Vaccine Damage Payment Act, 1979) in the UK and the National Childhood Vaccine Injury Compensation Programme (see National Childhood Vaccine Injury Act, 1986) in the US. As Kirkland (2016) shows, the introduction of the latter (and the emergence of the special 'vaccine court' that it adjudicates on), created a meeting place for the many epistemic communities interested in vaccine injury claims in the US. Its development reflected arguments made by the pharmaceutical industry that the usual process of civil litigation was creating unsustainable costs leading to vaccine manufacturing being unprofitable—which, at best, would mean rising prices and at worst harm to the supply of vaccines. Indeed, in 1984 one of the three manufacturers of the DTP combination vaccine announced it would stop making it, with a second considering leaving the market because of concerns about rising costs of liability insurance. Though manufacturers may have overstated their vulnerability to civil litigation, there was a growing sense of unease in vaccine supply. This, alongside some creative politicking within in the US government and the acknowledgement of the uncertain and precarious nature of civil litigation for parents of children harmed by vaccines was fundamental in the National Childhood Vaccine Injury Act passing into law in 1986 (see the work of Kirkland, 2016 for further detail).

New biotechnological innovations for making vaccines also developed (including the ability to genetically engineer vaccines). New and small biotechnology companies often possessed this new expertise rather than the larger, and older pharmaceutical companies, and thus pharmaceutical giants began purchasing smaller companies to gain access to new expertise. Under neoliberal conditions, intellectual property protection through vaccine patents became increasingly possible and desirable and this made vaccine development a more attractive field.[5] In this regard, patent protection essentially served to reconfigure vaccine knowledge as 'intellectual property' (Blume & Baylac-Paouly, 2021), and since the mid-2000s, a small pool of large vaccine developers/producers have been in competition globally including the well-known names of GlaxoSmithK-line, Merck and Pfizer (Reich, 2016, p. 7; see also Blume & Zanders, 2006, pp. 1826–1827).

---

[5] There is some debate about whether patent protection of intellectual property rights is harmful to the global distribution of vaccines. Charities, social justice campaigners and even the Director-General of the WHO have argued that vaccines could be made 'open source' and the underpinning technology and expertise shared freely so that vaccines can be produced cheaply in the places that need them. The other side of the argument, espoused by pharmaceutical companies and the Gates Foundation, is that the production of vaccines requires considerable manufacturing capacity, rigid quality assurance and regulatory processes which prevent the easy, risk-free production of vaccines globally. This debate was thrust into public consciousness by the COVID-19 crisis (see Wise, 2022).

As neoliberalism—with its ideological insistence on the benefits of the free market—became the dominant political ideology in western nations in the 1980s, the nature of vaccine development, changed as knowledge became increasingly proprietary. Blume and Baylac-Paouly (2021) show that the Bayh-Dole Act in the USA even went so far as to require scientists who had received government funding to commercialise their work and make it available to industry—which was done through scientists working in universities moving to or establishing the new, small biotech firms noted above. In this regard, the emerging neoliberal consensus interacted with scientific technological development to ensure that private companies held a central role in the composition of the immunisation social order.

With neoliberalism sweeping the globe in the 1980s and 1990s, private commercial interests increasingly diverged from the most pressing needs of global public health limiting the scope and success of the immunisation social order. For example, there was limited commercial interest in developing a vaccine for malaria (a disease predominantly affecting low-income countries where profit would be smaller). It thus became necessary to induce and incentivise profit-driven corporations to co-operate with the public sector to meet global public health needs. In this regard, global public-private partnerships emerged with the aim of encouraging the development of vaccines needed in low- and middle-income countries as well as facilitating access to vaccines. One such example was the Children's Vaccine Initiative (established in 1990 and which ultimately failed because of donor disagreements) (see Caddell, 1997). The Global Alliance for Vaccines and Immunization (known as Gavi, the Vaccine Alliance[6]), was subsequently founded in 2000 at the World Economic Forum to fulfil this role.

2.5.1   Vaccines and Autism

Sociologists of risk have argued that new types of risk (and understandings of risk) are generated by late modern societies, that society is (re)organised in response to risk and that new forms of behaviour emerge in response to risk (see Lupton, 1999 for an overview of the different theoretical approaches to risk). These sociocultural trends were evident in

[6] See Gavi.org.

the purported link between autism and vaccines. In 1998, the prestigious medical journal, the *Lancet*, published a study suggesting a link between the combined MMR vaccine and autism (Wakefield et al., 1998). The group of physicians writing the article hypothesised, based on children that they had treated, that the MMR vaccine produced gastrointestinal issues which they linked with autism. Just before the article was published, the lead author of the publication, Andrew Wakefield, held a press conference in which he announced the findings of the research. Although the paper did not assert causality, he called for the suspension of the MMR vaccine pending more research. This led to substantial media coverage and a fall in vaccination rates in the UK (Godlee et al., 2011). By 2004, the majority of the study's authors had renounced the research and ultimately the paper was retracted by the journal in 2010. It was also revealed that Wakefield had received money from legal firms seeking evidence to use to sue pharmaceutical companies—a conflict of interest that Wakefield did not declare and that ultimately help create what became a severe threat to the immunisation social order.

When vaccines controversies have been discussed in the public realm in the years since the MMR controversy, the narrative has predominantly focused on Andrew Wakefield rather than, for example, a parallel controversy in the USA concerning alleged connections between vaccine preservative thimerosal[7] (a compound which contains mercury) and autism that ultimately led to the removal of thimerosal from childhood vaccines (see Baker, 2008). Conis (2017) suggests that though the thimerosal controversy received a high degree of media and public attention at the time, this could not last because it was an inconvenient story for health authorities and ultimately posed a challenge to the immunisation social order (in Chapter 4 we return to the role played by the media in this example). Vaccine-sceptics could use it as 'confirmation' of their belief that vaccines have caused 'harm' or 'pose danger'. In contrast, the MMR controversy with a cultural narrative starring Wakefield, his misconduct and misinformed parents believing in a disproven theory is socially productive for health authorities. The story of the MMR controversy "affirms that vaccination is strictly a medical matter; that it works

---

[7] The FDA consulted vaccine experts, and large-scale studies concluded that there was no causal relationship between thimerosal and autism. However, with the possible connection between vaccines and autism firmly rooted in the mind of parents, thimerosal was removed from the childhood vaccines in the US as a precaution (Reich, 2016: 62–64).

when parents trust in experts; and that it is without risk or consequence—that there are no issues related to vaccination worthy of discussion beyond the matter raised by Wakefield and subsequently settled by a consensus of scientists" (Conis, 2017, pp. 305–306). In this sense, the MMR controversy and its retelling as both a cautionary tale and as evidence of the safety of vaccines by health authorities ultimately works to uphold rather than challenge the immunisation social order.

2.6   Conclusion

Beginning with Jesty, Jenner and smallpox and concluding in the neoliberal era, this chapter has charted the social stories at the centre of the history of vaccinology. We have sought to introduce the reader to the ways in which social and political forces have shaped the history of vaccines, vaccinology and the development of the immunisation social order. Vaccines as a technology, and their associated public health infrastructure, did not emerge from a social vacuum; the social, political and economic arrangements of the day and the interests and relationships between powerful actors have shaped the nature of vaccine innovation and utilisation. Our focus in this chapter has also enabled us to draw out challenges to the (emerging) immunisation social order and restrictions on its effective functioning (for example, the growing divergence between the needs of public health and private corporate interests under neoliberal conditions and the range of interests and social values influencing the nature and extent of vaccine controversy).

In the chapters that follow, we turn to examine more recent evidence of the salience of the social and political nature and impacts of vaccines and the functioning of the immunisation social order. We begin that endeavour with consideration of the importance of social values, politics and power relations within vaccine development and regulation.

References

Bailey, I. (2011). Edward Jenner, benefactor to mankind. In S. A. Plotkin (Ed.), *History of vaccine development* (pp. 21–25). Springer.

Baker, J. P. (2003). The pertussis vaccine controversy in Great Britain, 1974–1986. *Vaccine, 21*(25–26), 4003–4010. https://doi.org/10.1016/S0264-410X(03)00302-5

Baker, J. P. (2008). Mercury, vaccines, and autism: One controversy, three histories. *American Journal of Public Health, 98*(2), 244–253.

Baxby, D. (2011). Edward Jenner's role in the introduction of smallpox vaccine. In S. A. Plotkin (Ed.), *History of vaccine development* (pp. 13–19) Springer.

Bazin, H. (2011) Pasteur and the birth of vaccines made in the laboratory. In S. A. Plotkin (Ed.), *History of vaccine development* (pp. 33–45). Springer.

BBC News (2021). Benjamin Jesty: The unsung hero of vaccination. https://www.bbc.co.uk/news/uk-england-dorset-57460445

Blume, S. (2017). *Immunization: How vaccines became controversial.* Reaktion Books.

Blume, S., & Baylac-Paouly, B. (2021). Introduction. In S. Blume & B. Baylac-Paouly (Eds.), *Immunization and states: The politics of making vaccines* (pp. 1–19). Routledge.

Blume, S., & Zanders, M. (2006). Vaccine independence, local competences and globalisation: Lessons from the history of pertussis vaccines. *Social Science & Medicine, 63*(7), 1825–1835. https://doi.org/10.1016/j.socscimed.2006.04.014

Bryder, L. (1999). 'We shall not find salvation in inoculation': BCG vaccination in Scandinavia, Britain and the USA, 1921–1960. *Social Science & Medicine, 49*(9), 1157–1167. https://doi.org/10.1016/S0277-9536(99)00157-4

Caddell, A. (1997). The children's vaccine initiative. *Africa Health, 20*(1), 15.

Calnan, M., & Douglass, T. (2020). Hopes, hesitancy and the risky business of vaccine development. *Health, Risk & Society, 22*(5–6), 291–304. https://doi.org/10.1080/13698575.2020.1846687

Carapetis, J. R. (2006). The Cutter incident: How America's first polio vaccine led to the growing vaccine crisis. *BMJ, 332*(7543), 733.

Colgrove, J. (2006). *State of immunity: The politics of vaccination in twentieth century America.* University of California Press.

Conis, E. (2017). Vaccines, pesticides, and narratives of exposure and evidence. *Canadian Bulletin of Medical History, 34*(2), 297–326. https://doi.org/10.3138/cbmh.190-21122016

Dubé, E., Vivion, M., & MacDonald, N. E. (2015). Vaccine hesitancy, vaccine refusal and the anti-vaccine movement: Influence, impact and implications. *Expert Review of Vaccines, 14*(1), 99–117. https://doi.org/10.1586/14760584.2015.964212

Durbach, N. (2005). *Bodily matters: The anti-vaccination movement in England, 1853–1907.* Duke University Press.

Esparza, J., Lederman, S., Nitsche, A., & Damaso, C. R. (2020). Early smallpox vaccine manufacturing in the United States: Introduction of the "animal vaccine" in 1870, establishment of "vaccine farms", and the beginnings of the vaccine industry. *Vaccine, 38*(30), 4773–4779. https://doi.org/10.1016/j.vaccine.2020.05.037

Godlee, F., Smith, J., & Marcovitch, H. (2011). Wakefield's article linking MMR vaccine and autism was fraudulent. *BMJ*, *342*. https://doi.org/10.1136/bmj.c7452

Horton, R. (1995). Myths in medicine. Jenner did not discover vaccination. *BMJ*, *310*(6971), 62. https://doi.org/10.1136/bmj.310.6971.62a

Hotez, P. J. (2017). Russian–United States vaccine science diplomacy: Preserving the legacy. *PLoS Neglected Tropical Diseases, 11*(5), https://doi.org/10.1371/journal.pntd.0005320

Kirkland, A. (2016). *Vaccine court: The law and politics of injury*. NYU Press.

Kulenkampff, M., Schwartzman, J. S., & Wilson, J. (1974). Neurological complications of pertussis inoculation. *Archives of Disease in Childhood, 49*(1), 46–49.

Latour, B. (1993). *The pasteurization of France*. Harvard University Press.

Leung, A. K. C. (2011). "Variolation" and vaccination in late imperial China, ca 1570–1911. In *History of vaccine* development (pp. 5–12). Springer.

Löwy, I. (1994). On hybridizations, networks and new disciplines: The Pasteur Institute and the development of microbiology in France. *Studies in History and Philosophy of Science Part A, 25*(5), 655–688. https://doi.org/10.1016/0039-3681(94)90035-3

Luca, S., & Mihaescu, T. (2013). History of BCG vaccine. *Maedica, 8*(1), 53–58.

Lupton, D. (1999). *Risk and sociocultural theory: New directions and perspectives*. Cambridge University Press.

Manela, E. (2010). A pox on your narrative: Writing disease control into Cold War history. *Diplomatic History, 34*(2), 299–323. https://doi.org/10.1111/j.1467-7709.2009.00850.x

Offit, P. A. (2005). The Cutter incident, 50 years later. *New England Journal of Medicine, 352*(14), 1411–1412. https://doi.org/10.1056/NEJMp048180

Oshinsky, D. M. (2005). *Polio: An American story*. Oxford University Press.

Pead, P. J. (2006). Benjamin Jesty: The first vaccinator revealed. *The Lancet, 368*(9554), 2202. https://doi.org/10.1016/S0140-6736(06)69878-4

Pead, P. J. (2017a). *The Homespun origins of vaccination: A brief history*. Vivlia Limited.

Pead, P. J. (2017b). Vaccination's forgotten origins. *Pediatrics, 139*(4). https://doi.org/10.1542/peds.2016-2833

Pead, P. J. (2019). *Benjamin Jesty, the Grandfather of Vaccination*. Cambridge Scholars Publishing.

Plotkin, S. A., & Plotkin, S. L. (2011). The development of vaccines: How the past led to the future. *Nature Reviews Microbiology, 9*(12), 889–893.

Poland, G. A., & Jacobson, R. M. (2001). Understanding those who do not understand: A brief review of the anti-vaccine movement. *Vaccine, 19*(17–19), 2440–2445. https://doi.org/10.1016/S0264-410X(00)00469-2

Poland, G. A., & Jacobson, R. M. (2011). The age-old struggle against the antivaccinationists. *New England Journal of Medicine, 364*(2), 97–99.

Reagan, L. J. (2012). *Dangerous pregnancies: Mothers, disabilities, and abortion in modern America.* University of California Press.

Reich, J. A. (2016). *Calling the shots.* New York University Press.

Riedel, S. (2005). Edward Jenner and the history of smallpox and vaccination. *Baylor University Medical Center Proceedings, 18*(1), 21–25. https://doi.org/10.1080/08998280.2005.11928028

Smith, K. A. (2012). Louis Pasteur, the father of immunology? *Frontiers in Immunology, 3,* 68. https://doi.org/10.3389/fimmu.2012.00068

Stern, A. M., & Markel, H. (2005). The history of vaccines and immunization: Familiar patterns, new challenges. *Health Affairs, 24*(3), 611–621. https://doi.org/10.1377/hlthaff.24.3.611

Wakefield, A. J., Murch, S. H., Anthony, A., Linnell, J., Casson, D. M., Malik, M., Berelowitz, M., Dhillon, A. P., Thomson, M. A., Harvey, P., Valentine, A., Davies, S. E., & Walker-Smith, J. A. (1998). RETRACTED: Ileal-lymphoid-nodular hyperplasia, non-specific colitis, and pervasive developmental disorder in children. *The Lancet, 351*(9103), 637–641. https://doi.org/10.1016/s0140-6736(97)11096-0

Wise, J. (2022). Covid-19: Drug companies urged to share vaccine technology to boost equity and access. *BMJ, 377.* https://doi.org/10.1136/bmj.o1086

CHAPTER 3

Values, Politics and Power Relations in the Development and Regulation of Vaccines

Abstract Here we begin our substantive exploration of the modern social and political nature and impacts of vaccines. We do so by examining examples of how subjective values, social relationships, power and interests influence and reshape the interconnected processes of development and regulation. First, the chapter begins with an overview of the central actors and processes in the development and regulatory assessment of vaccines. In doing this, we discuss the process of testing vaccine candidates (a crucial component in the immunisation social order and its maintenance) and the nature of the global vaccine market. Following this, we turn to examine vaccines as political entities discussing how gendered and heteronormative values were reflected in and (re)shaped by the development and initial response to the first HPV vaccine. The chapter also analyses the political nature of vaccines in relation to the pharmaceutical turn in national security. Next, the chapter looks at the case of the first vaccine developed to prevent rotavirus. This discussion highlights the significance of social values in regulatory assessment and the withdrawal of the vaccine from the market. Finally, the chapter explores the relations between powerful actors in the development and regulation of COVID-19 vaccines.

Keywords Vaccine Development and Regulation · Politics · Social Values · Power · COVID-19 Vaccines

© The Author(s), under exclusive license to Springer Nature Switzerland AG 2024
T. Douglass and A. Anderson, *Vaccines in Society*,
https://doi.org/10.1007/978-3-031-61269-5_3

3.1   Introduction

Vaccine development and regulation may initially appear to be of limited interest to or outside of the analytical expertise of social scientists. However, as medical sociology, and science and technology studies in particular show us, science and medicine are inherently and fundamentally social phenomena. Medical technologies emerging from scientific research are not in some sense separate from or outside the society in which they are developed—social and political conditions profoundly affect scientific processes and technology in many ways (see Collins & Pinch, 1993; MacKenzie & Wajcman, 1999; Sismondo, 2004). Indeed, Casper and Carpenter (2008) show that the development of vaccines not only occurs within and is impacted by a particular social and political context but also interacts with and reshapes the social and political milieu. In other words, vaccine development and regulation (as the initial stages of the 'pharmaceutical life course' discussed in Chapter 1) reveal and/or activate social and political values, relations, controversies which are embedded in, or which present a problem or challenge to the immunisation social order.

This chapter begins our substantive exploration of the modern social and political nature and impacts of vaccines. It does so by examining examples of how subjective values, social relationships, power and interests influence and reshape the interconnected processes of development and regulation. First, the chapter begins with an overview of the central actors and processes in the development and regulatory assessment of vaccines. In doing this we discuss the process of testing vaccine candidates (a crucial component in the immunisation social order and its maintenance) and the nature of the global vaccine market. Following this we turn to examine vaccines as political entities discussing how gendered and heteronormative values were reflected in and (re)shaped by the development and initial response to HPV vaccines. The chapter also analyses the political nature of vaccines in relation to the pharmaceutical turn in national security. Next, the chapter looks at the case of RotaShield, the first vaccine developed to prevent rotavirus. This discussion highlights the significance of social values in regulatory assessment and the withdrawal of the vaccine from the market. Finally, the chapter explores the relations between powerful actors in the development of COVID-19 vaccines and discusses the role played by interests in shaping the approach to and nature of the processes of their development and regulatory assessment.

3.2   ACTORS, PROCESSES

Before turning to the substantive examples of values, relations and interests shaping or being reshaped by vaccine development, it is necessary to lay out the actors and processes central to developing and manufacturing vaccines. This will begin to illuminate the social, political and economic context that vaccine development and regulation occurs within, as well as some central relationships and the interests of powerful actors. Some of the vaccines used globally to protect people against a range of dangerous and debilitating disease have been in existence for many years as discussed in the previous chapter, however the work of developing and producing new vaccines (as well as manufacturing established vaccines) involves pharmaceutical and biotechnology companies sometimes in collaboration with public sector institutions, universities and non-governmental organisations.

Vaccine development is a difficult enterprise (Calnan & Douglass, 2020). Indeed, only 6% of vaccines that begin development successfully reach the market. It takes many years to successfully develop a vaccine, but in less economically favourable contexts it often takes much longer. For example, in the case of Ebola Virus Disease, which predominantly affects Western and sub-Saharan countries, it took more than 40 years for a vaccine to complete development (Calnan & Douglass, 2020; Mullard, 2020). Despite lengthy development timelines, recent figures suggest that the global vaccine market is worth $141 billion; this has dramatically risen from a valuation of $38 billion in 2019 (which was before the pandemic and the associated development and global roll out of the COVID-19 vaccines) (WHO, 2022). To demonstrate the sheer comparative size and value of the vaccine market in relation to other crucial pharmaceutical products, the oncology drugs market was valued around $138 billion[1] in 2022 while the cardiovascular disease drugs market was worth $144 billion[2] in 2023.

The importance of profit in the private sector means that commercial and public health interests do not always align (see Blume & Baylac-Paouly, 2021). Funding provided by state, supranational and non-governmental organisations is an important driver of research, particularly for vaccines targeting the most pressing public health problems in the

[1] See https://www.precedenceresearch.com/cardiovascular-drugs-market.

[2] See https://www.precedenceresearch.com/cancer-drugs-market and.

least developed countries. In one example, the Canadian government committed $7 million to fund research into an Ebola vaccine for the purposes of biodefence (Strauss, 2014). In other examples, the European Commission, prior to the COVID-19 pandemic, provided €650 million for vaccine and vaccination research and innovation through its Horizon 2020 funding programme in the years 2014–2020 (Florio et al., 2023). It provided another €350 million to fund COVID-19 vaccine development. Furthermore, the Gates Foundation, a philanthropic endeavour founded by one of the world's richest people, Bill Gates, has provided billions of dollars to fund vaccine research, distribution and access globally.[3] In a final example, as will be discussed later in this chapter, 97% of the funding shaping directly or indirectly the development of the Oxford-AstraZeneca vaccine was provided by non-commercial sources (Cross et al., 2021).

When developing a vaccine, the process typically involves distinct stages of pre-clinical and clinical trials (see Gilbert & Green, 2021; Weijer, 2020). These data are then submitted to regulatory authorities—such as the Medicines and Healthcare products Regulatory Authority (MHRA) in Britain, The Food and Drug Administration (FDA) in the USA or the European Medicines Agency (EMA)—who assess evidence of efficacy, safety and quality.

The initial stage of testing involves pre-clinical and toxicology studies using animals to check that a candidate vaccine provokes an immune response and is safe. This initial work helps to attract funding and is required to proceed to the next stage of the process involving testing the candidate vaccine on humans. Subsequently, there are three phases of clinical trials. Phase I trials test the candidate vaccine on a small number of healthy human participants with a particular focus on safety. Phase II trials are concerned with immune response and safety, this time involving hundreds of participants and providing more substantial evidence of safety and efficacy. Phase III trials compare the candidate vaccine against placebo or other best-available intervention. This takes place at a much broader level, with many different types of people taking part in the trial totalling

---

[3] It is worth noting that a range of groups with different interests contest the influence of the Gates Foundation on global public health. This includes activists who oppose vaccination. It also includes supporters of vaccination who are concerned with the problematic political and ethical dimensions of global access to vaccines, intellectual property rights and for-profit models of vaccine production, as well as the arguably undemocratic role of wealthy philanthropists.

thousands or tens of thousands. This phase is constructed to provide well-powered statistical evidence about whether a vaccine works, as well as evidence about uncommon and rare side effects.

After the three phases of clinical trials, post-marketing surveillance (known as pharmacovigilance) monitors previously unidentified adverse effects once vaccines are in use (often thought of as Phase IV). For example, the MHRA runs the Yellow Card scheme which collects and monitors information on safety concerns. This relies on the vaccinated public, parents and healthcare professionals for reports of adverse events. Finally, new vaccines may also be evaluated by health authorities in public health terms (with a focus on which populations should be vaccinated) and by health economists in the terms of cost-effectiveness (the expected health benefit in relation to the cost of an intervention).

3.3   Vaccines as Political Artefacts

3.3.1   Gender Norms, Heteronormativity and the HPV Vaccine

Social and political values are embedded in vaccine development and, in turn, these sociotechnical entities reshape social and political values across the life course of these products. Social research concerned with the initial development of HPV vaccines demonstrates these dynamics (Carpenter & Casper, 2009; Casper & Carpenter, 2008). Although HPV may also cause penile, anal and throat cancers the initial development, testing and licensing in the USA of HPV vaccination targeted cervical cancer (as caused by the sexual transmission of HPV) in women. As such, HPV vaccines were feminised at their inception[4] (Daley et al., 2017). This both reflected and worked to reinforce the widespread cultural understanding of sexual health as a 'women's issue' (Carpenter & Casper, 2009).

When the first HPV vaccine was introduced in the mid-2000s, a narrative developed alongside it as the 'promiscuity vaccine'. This argument, emerging primarily from conservative elements[5] in US society, suggested (without evidence) that the vaccine would encourage promiscuity among

---

[4] It is only in more recent years that the HPV vaccine has been offered to boys, beginning in 2019 in the UK.

[5] There is also evidence that some medical professionals were less likely to recommend the vaccine if they believed that administering the HPV vaccine increased the chances of unprotected sexual activity in adolescents (Suryadevara et al., 2015).

teenage girls because of the lower threat of disease caused by HPV, such as cervical cancer. This specific cultural reaction to the introduction of the HPV vaccine, argue Carpenter and Casper (2009), was shaped by understandings of gender and sexuality, while also helping to reconfigure some of these cultural notions (usefully highlighting the intersection of social values and a new vaccine). These authors compare the introduction of the HPV vaccine to debates about the value of male circumcision as a preventative measure against HIV transmission. In contrast to the development of the HPV vaccine, and despite both technologies having preventative sexual health intentions, the scientific and societal conversations about male circumcision did not lead to increased anxiety about the sexual activities of teenage boys. The authors argue that this reflects gendered notions of sexuality where girls (or women) are viewed as either innocent or fallen, and boys (or men) as inherently sexually driven. At the same time, the development of the HPV vaccine led to an increased cultural sensitivity to the (eventual) sexual activity and availability of girls and young women—simply because the vaccine protects against a virus which is transmitted via sexual intercourse. Overall, HPV vaccine is an example not only of gender norms being embedded in vaccine development and thus the nature of the immunisation social order, but also how vaccine development can reshape political and cultural values and animate controversies.

Furthermore, Daley et al. (2017) show how the initial logic underpinning the licensing and use of HPV vaccines reflected a different set of social and political values. Alongside its gendered nature, the development, testing and deployment of HPV vaccines (and thus the immunisation social order) were also initially embedded with heteronormativity. Men who engage in sexual relationships with other men are at higher risk of HPV-related outcomes. However, those vaccinated against HPV have a lower risk of developing anal cancer. Due to the heteronormative logic of the HPV vaccine built into the development, testing and usage of the original vaccine, this group of men were ignored and did not initially receive the protection offered by the HPV vaccine.[6] In this sense, social and political values initially restricted optimal levels of vaccine coverage harming the immunisation social order.

---

[6] In 2018 men up to the age of 45 became eligible for free HPV vaccination provided by the NHS.

3.3.2 National Security

In a very different example, analysis offered through the lens of international relations and security studies suggests that vaccines—and pharmaceutical products more generally—are also political objects in terms of their use in national security and defence. Political concern about global health security has grown in significance since the early 2000s. Since this time, governments have increasingly wrestled with the question of how to protect their citizens and economies against the twin health security threats of emerging infectious disease and bioterrorism. As Elbe (2014; see also 2018) discusses, predating the COVID-19 pandemic, government awareness of threats to national and global health security have been tied to increasing interest in developing and strengthening pharmaceutical defences. In this regard, governments have sought to protect their populations through investment in the development and stockpiling of medical countermeasures which are pharmaceutical interventions—including (though not limited to) vaccines—that can be deployed in the event of an emerging natural or terrorist threat to health security. This is a clear example of what Anderson (2010, p. 792) calls 'anticipatory action'; this is the "means through which life in contemporary liberal democracies is secured, conducted, disciplined and normalised". In this sense, the future is made present and thus precautionary or preparative action becomes a necessary cause.

Elbe (2014, p. 928) states that "[w]hat is arguably a country's highest political priority—ensuring national security—is now closely dependent upon a government's ability not just to actively develop and acquire, but also to stockpile and rapidly disseminate, large volumes of medical countermeasures". National security priorities are thus embedded in and help construct the immunisation social order in capitalist countries. The pharmaceutical turn in security, or the pharmaceuticalisation of security, reflects a more general trend with origins in the 1980s of the growing significance within everyday life of a molecular, biomedical knowledge (Rose, 2007a, 2007b) and the increasing power of biomedical actors, such as the pharmaceutical industry, to influence the societies in which we live (see Douglass & Calnan, 2022 for a more focused discussion of the conceptual side of this literature).

As Elbe shows (2014), the molecular version of life propagated by biomedical actors has created new anxieties and insecurities about the possible harm caused by terroristic manipulation at the molecular level as well as concerns about mutating viruses and bacteria found in nature. In response, a vast investment (both by the private sector and governments) in the development of new pharmaceutical products to defend or strengthen health security has occurred, as well as adapting regulatory environments to be facilitative of innovation and to enable pharmaceutical countermeasures to be widely and speedily available as the immunisation social order is reconstructed and reimagined. Indeed, the European Medicines Agency (EMA) introduced three procedures designed to increase regulatory flexibility and speed up the assessment of influenza vaccines in the event of a pandemic to make them available for use more quickly. The three procedures introduced include, the first, a mock-up procedure, which enables a vaccine to be authorised in advance based on an influenza strain that could possibly cause a pandemic. Second, an emergency procedure, which reduces the regulatory timeline by up to two-thirds. Finally, a modification procedure, meaning that a flu vaccine can be changed to provide protection against a pandemic strain of influenza. It is thought that these measures not only expedite the regulatory assessment of vaccines in a possible crisis, but also increase the likelihood of commercial investment in vaccine development for use in the European Union.

The pharmaceutical turn in national security has led to a political role for vaccines—imbuing vaccines (and other pharmaceutical products) with securing the safety and health of a state's citizens. It has also led to research into new types of pharmaceutical products (that otherwise, if not for political influence, would not occur) and has reshaped procedures for testing and assessing the safety and efficacy of vaccines. In this sense, the role of vaccines in national security reflects the broader biopolitical character of contemporary society where political authorities are engaged in the management of human existence (see Rose, 2001) through the (re)construction of the immunisation social order. Equally, ensuring uninterrupted economic functioning (or at least minimising disruption) through biomedical intervention is a central priority.

3.4   Social Values in Regulatory Assessment

The case of RotaShield, the first vaccine to protect against rotavirus (the most common global cause of severe diarrhoeal disease in infants and young children), reveals how social values connect and intersect with empirical evidence during regulatory decision-making about vaccines

(Schwartz, 2012). RotaShield was licensed by the Food and Drug Administration (FDA) on 31 August 1998. In the USA, though the FDA assesses safety and efficacy data, and thus licenses vaccines for use, the Centre for Disease Control (CDC) also has an important role. The CDC issues recommendations about which populations should receive vaccination. Drawing on the work of its Advisory Committee on Immunization Practices (ACIP), recommendations published by the CDC are viewed as vitally important to the commercial and medical success of a vaccine. RotaShield was officially recommended for all infants with three doses to be delivered at ages two, four and six months in early 1999. Importantly, the FDA and CDC also jointly run the Vaccine Adverse Event Reporting System (VAERS). As discussed earlier, this system allows patients, physicians or concerned third parties to report potential adverse effects linked to a vaccine. This system operates as an early warning signal for a possible vaccine safety problem. In the first quarter of 1999, there had been 62 reports of adverse events to VAERS. This included three reports of intussusception—an uncommon, though very serious condition where part of the intestine descends into a distal segment that is most common in infants in their first year of life—with nine more reports of intussusception by June 1999. As a result, pending an investigation, the CDC decided to temporarily suspend use of the vaccine in July 1999.

The CDC's decision to stop the use of RotaShield was framed in the language of epidemiology and with reference solely to the confirmed and quantified risk of intussusception and the significantly increased incidence of the condition following the vaccination. This is illustrated by the following quote:

> The Advisory Committee on Immunization Practices, after review of the currently available information from several sources, has concluded that intussusception occurs with significantly increased frequency in the first one to two weeks following vaccination... Therefore, the ACIP no longer recommends routine immunization of infants [with RotaShield]. (CDC 1999, pp. 178–79)

However, Schwartz (2012) shows that absent in the regulatory deliberation and public statements about the withdrawal of RotaShield from the market was clear comparison between the risks and benefits of the vaccine. All vaccines (and, indeed, pharmaceutical treatments more generally) have possible risks—with the RotaShield vaccine initially estimated to cause intussusception in one in 5000 cases, though it was later argued to be lower in frequency. However, there was no discussion of whether the vaccine had passed an unacceptable threshold for the frequency of adverse effects, nor was there mention of whether intussusception—a potentially fatal adverse effect—was inherently unacceptable despite the benefits of prevention in the population.

Several years after the withdrawal, and as other researchers began to challenge the association between the vaccine and the frequency of intussusception, CDC staff published a revised public rationale for the withdrawal. This revealed, Schwartz argues, the value judgements and social factors that influenced the CDC's decision-making (see Murphy et al., 2003). At the time the safety concerns about RotaShield were emerging, a much larger controversy about vaccine safety and necessity was taking place reflecting the suggestion of links between childhood vaccines and autism and the possible risk of thimerosal, a preservative containing mercury (see Chapter 2). Acknowledging these more general concerns about vaccines, as well as news media and political interest in the topic, the CDC emphasised in this later publication how their decision-making had considered the interests of the US childhood vaccination programme generally. In this context, continued use of RotaShield, a vaccine causing a possibly fatal adverse reaction in a significant portion of infants vaccinated could, as such, cause a collapse in public trust and support for vaccination generally. Indeed, Schwartz (2012, pp. 298–299) states

> [a] that quantitative threshold of acceptable risk was never identified for RotaShield, but a qualitative threshold was unmistakably passed. This threshold was not expressed in terms of disease prevented compared with intussusceptions caused but as a threshold reflecting political viability and public perception.

To be clear, the social dimensions of the decision to stop the use of RotaShield were not discussed at the time of the withdrawal. Instead, an ostensibly 'objective' epidemiological quantitative justification was used. It was only as challenges to the quantitative safety evidence occurred did the decision-making narrative shift to reveal the value judgements and importance of a social context of controversy about vaccines on the decision to withdraw RotaShield.

Schwartz (2012) additionally shows that there were global consequences associated with the decision to withdraw RotaShield from use in the USA. The CDC were aware that decision-making in the US might pre-empt regulatory decision-making in other parts of the world—including in developing countries with higher incidences of rotavirus—where the benefits might be more substantial and thus the balance of risk and benefit more favourable. Efficacy and safety data in developing countries were not available and thus regulatory decision-making in the US made the vaccine politically non-viable in other contexts. Though there were attempts to show that judgements in the US may not apply elsewhere, the impacts of the context at the time of the withdrawal and of subjective values present in US decision-making shaped the viability of the vaccine in other parts of the world. Health officials could not palatably deploy a vaccine in their own country deemed too unsafe for American children. Overall, the example of RotaShield provides a valuable example of how social values can influence the regulatory assessment of vaccines, their subsequent or continued use, as well as how the nature and functioning of the immunisation social order (domestically and internationally) can be reshaped and challenged by sociological forces.

3.5 Power Relations and Interests in the Development and Regulatory Assessment of COVID-19 Vaccines

Calnan and Douglass (2022) have sociologically analysed COVID-19 policymaking, and in the process, cast light on the power relations and interests embedded in vaccine development and regulation. They approach the healthcare sphere generally, and vaccine development and regulation specifically, as being comprised of several interest groups—including the government, commercial entities, such as the pharmaceutical industry, scientists and health professionals, and patients/the public—that contend for power and legitimacy and who attempt to assert their own priorities or vision of healthcare delivery (see Gabe et al., 2012). Importantly, this type of work requires analysis of the salience of both direct and indirect influences, interests and strategies on policymaking and policy outcomes relating to vaccine development and regulation. These authors also note the value of assessing if and how interest groups collaborate or build allegiances that enable or support policymaking and specific policy outcomes—which were some of the most important elements ulti-mately highlighted by their research (Calnan & Douglass, 2022). The approach taken by these authors variously reveals the following important elements: the relations between actors and the dynamics of power within the immunisation social order during the COVID-19 crisis as well as the importance of interests in shaping the approach to COVID-19 vaccine development and regulation.

State funding/taxpayer money was central to the research that ulti-mately led to the development of the Oxford-AstraZeneca vaccine (see DHSC, 2021). The UK government invested £120 million into various vaccine development projects between 2016 and 2021. This included £1.87 million awarded to the University of Oxford for the develop-ment of a MERS vaccine—revealing the importance of relationships between the state and scientific researchers within the immunisation social order. Oxford was awarded further funding in the early phases of the pandemic to repurpose their work to fight COVID-19 (House of Commons Health and Social Care and Science and Technology Committees, 2021). Furthermore, publicly funded research was more generally important to the development of the technology underpin-ning the Oxford-AstraZeneca vaccine (Cross et al., 2021). 97% of the funding (reaching hundreds of millions of pounds) contributing directly or indirectly to the technology came from government or charitable sources—such as the British and American governments, the European Commission, the Wellcome Trust and other scientific institutes. Compar-atively, less than 2% was provided by the pharmaceutical Industry (ibid). Here we can see that relationships between actors largely other than the pharmaceutical industry were central to the underpinning COVID-19 vaccine research—despite the dominant narrative attributing the success of the vaccine to 'capitalism' and commercial 'greed' (Allegretti & Elgot, 2021) rather than scientific research funded by non-commercial actors.

Despite the considerable investment in COVID-19 vaccine research, there were no guarantees that the vaccines being developed to protect people against COVID-19 would be effective or sufficiently safe when they were tested. On the other hand, considering the rising death and lockdown restrictions impacting social and economic life during the first year of the pandemic in 2020, should a safe and effective vaccine be successfully developed, the government in Westminster and the Vaccine Taskforce (VTF) (formed in April 2020 to support COVID-19 vaccine research and manufacture) wanted to be able to quickly begin vaccinating the most vulnerable people. As a result, the government agreed 'at risk' contracts with some manufacturers for the supply of a range of COVID-19 vaccines (DHSC, 2021). These contracts meant that the manufacture of COVID-19 vaccines could begin before the three phases of clinical trials and regulatory approval had been given—and thus the government could be ready to start the vaccination programme immediately upon regulatory authorisation (ibid). This meant that the state rather than commercial entities absorbed the risk of beginning to manufacture vaccines despite the possibility that the vaccines would ultimately not be confirmed by the regulatory body, the MHRA, to be safe and/or effective (though they were). The pharmaceutical industry exerted its substantial power and influence, leveraging the need for its manufacturing expertise and capacity to agree favourable terms with the government particularly in terms of establishing a financially de-risked role in development and manufacturing. The financial risk of the development and manufacturing was therefore substantially greater for the government than for the pharmaceutical industry. However, perhaps reflecting the crisis circumstances in particular, the government was willing to accept the financial risk to protect public health and the economy, and it ultimately served the government's objectives and interests as well as leading to financial and reputational gains for some pharmaceutical companies (thus serving the pharmaceutical industry's commercial interests).

In terms of the relationships between powerful actors tasked with responding to the COVID-19 crisis, it is important to understand that the regulation of COVID-19 vaccines was distinctive—it differed from the traditional model of testing pharmaceutical products outlined earlier in this chapter. In an expedited manner, the MHRA reviewed the trial data on a rolling basis rather than receiving all data at the end of the three phases of trials as would normally occur (DHSC, 2021). In this regard, the government, the regulator and the pharmaceutical industry operated together in a unique alliance in the development and regulation of COVID-19 vaccines to enable the COVID-19 vaccination programme to begin as soon as possible—ultimately leading to relatively high levels of vaccine take-up, vulnerable lives saved and eventually allowing for lockdown restrictions on social and economic life to be lifted.

3.6   CONCLUSION

This chapter has revealed how vaccine development and regulatory activity can be influenced and reshaped by social and political forces. In other words, we have shown that vaccine development and regulation (as the initial stages of the 'pharmaceutical life course') reveal and/ or activate social and political values, relations, controversies embedded in or as challenging the immunisation social order. Following a brief exploration of the central actors and processes in the development and regulation of vaccines, this chapter has offered several case studies. We began with an exploration of how the initial public reaction to the HPV vaccine was shaped by social and political values but also how values were embedded in and subsequently reshaped by its development. Embedded gender norms and heteronormativity restricted vaccine coverage and thus the optimal functioning of the immunisation social order. Furthermore, we explored how the pharmaceutical turn in national security has politically imbued vaccines with securing the health and safety of a state's citizens, how this turn has led to new types of pharmaceutical products and how it has introduced new procedures for testing and assessing the safety and efficacy of vaccines and thus the nature and functioning of the immunisation social order. In another example, despite health authorities initially providing an epidemiological justification, we demonstrated the centrality of social values in and contextual nature of regulatory decision-making and the subsequent withdrawal of the first rotavirus vaccine in the USA. Finally, focusing on the development and regulation of COVID-19 vaccines in Britain, we analysed the relations, power dynamics and impacts of the interests of powerful groups within the immunisation social order.

REFERENCES

Allegretti, A., & Elgot, J. (2021) Covid: 'Greed' and capitalism behind vaccine success, Johnson tells MPs. *The Guardian*. https://www.theguardian.com/politics/2021/mar/23/greed-and-capitalism-behind-jabsuccess-boris-johnson-tells-mps

Anderson, B. (2010). Pre-emption, precaution, preparedness: Anticipatory action and future geographies. *Progress in Human Geography, 34*(6), 777–798. https://doi.org/10.1177/0309132510362600

Blume, S., & Baylac-Paouly, B. (2021). Introduction. In S. Blume & B. Baylac-Paouly (Eds.), *Immunization and states: The politics of making vaccines* (pp. 1–19). Routledge.

Calnan, M., & Douglass, T. (2020). Hopes, hesitancy and the risky business of vaccine development. *Health, Risk & Society, 22*(5–6), 291–304. https://doi.org/10.1080/13698575.2020.1846687

Calnan, M., & Douglass, T. (2022) *Power, policy and the pandemic: A sociological analysis of COVID-19 policy in England.* Emerald Publishing Limited.

Collins, H., & Pinch, T. (1993) *The Golem: What everyone should know about science.* Cambridge University Press.

Carpenter, L. M., & Casper, M. J. (2009). A tale of two technologies: HPV vaccination, male circumcision, and sexual health. *Gender & Society, 23*(6), 790–816. https://doi.org/10.1177/0891243209352490

Casper, M. J., & Carpenter, L. M. (2008). Sex, drugs, and politics: The HPV vaccine for cervical cancer. *Sociology of Health & Illness, 30*(6), 886–899. https://doi.org/10.1111/j.1467-9566.2008.01100.x

CDC (Centers for Disease Control and Prevention) (1999, October 22). Advisory Committee on Immunization Practices meeting. Transcript.

Cross, S., Rho, Y., Reddy, H., Pepperrell, T., Rodgers, F., Osborne, R., Eni-Olotu, A., Banerjee, R., Wimmer, S., & Keestra, S. (2021) Who funded the research behind the Oxford–AstraZeneca COVID-19 vaccine?. *BMJ Global Health, 6*(12), e007321. https://doi.org/10.1136/bmjgh-2021-007321

Daley, E. M., Vamos, C. A., Thompson, E. L., Zimet, G. D., Rosberger, Z., Merrell, L., & Kline, N. S. (2017). The feminization of HPV: How science, politics, economics and gender norms shaped US HPV vaccine implementation. *Papillomavirus Research, 3*, 142–148. https://doi.org/10.1016/j.pvr.2017.04.004

DHSC. (2021). *UK COVID-19 vaccines delivery plan.* https://assets.publishing.service.gov.uk/government/uploads/system/uploads/attachment_data/file/951928/uk-covid-19-vaccines-delivery-plan-final.pdf

Douglass, T., & Calnan, M. (2022) Medicalisation and pharmaceuticalisation: A conceptual analysis. In S.Scrimshaw, S. Lane, J. Fisher & R. Rubinstein (Eds.), *The sage handbook of social studies of health and medicine.* Sage. Chapter 25.

Elbe, S. (2014). The pharmaceuticalisation of security: Molecular biomedicine, antiviral stockpiles, and global health security. *Review of International Studies, 40*(5), 919–938. https://doi.org/10.1017/S0260210514000151

Elbe, S. (2018). *Pandemics, pills, and politics: Governing global health security.* John Hopkins University Press.

Florio, M., Gamba, S., Pancotti, C., Cisco, G., & Gazzo, M. (2023). *Mapping of long-term public and private investments in the development of COVID-19 vaccines.* https://www.europarl.europa.eu/RegData/etudes/STUD/2023/740072/IPOL_STU(2023)740072_EN.pdf

Gabe, J., Chamberlain, K., Norris, P., Dew, K., Madden, H., & Hodgetts, D. (2012). The debate about the funding of Herceptin: A case study of 'countervailing powers.' *Social Science & Medicine, 75*(12), 2353–2361. https://doi.org/10.1016/j.socscimed.2012.09.009

Gilbert, S., & Green, C. (2021). *Vaxxers: The inside story of the Oxford AstraZeneca Vaccine and the race against the virus.* Hodder and Stoughton.

House of Commons Health and Social Care and Science and Technology Committees. (2021) *Sixth report of the health and social care committee and third report of the science and technology committee of session 2021–2022.* https://committees.parliament.uk/publications/7496/documents/78687/default/

MacKenzie, D., & Wajcman, J. (1999). *The social shaping of technology.* Open University Press.

Mullard, A. (2020). FDA approves antibody cocktail for Ebola virus. *Nature Reviews Drug Discovery, 19*(12), 827–828.

Murphy, T., Smith, P., Gargiullo, P., & Schwartz, B. (2003). The first rotavirus vaccine and intussusception: Epidemiological studies and policy decisions. *Journal of Infectious Diseases, 187*, 1309–1313.

Rose, N. (2001). The politics of life itself. *Theory, Culture & Society, 18*(6), 1–30. https://doi.org/10.1177/02632760122052020

Rose, N. (2007a). Beyond medicalisation. *The Lancet, 369*(9562), 700–702. https://doi.org/10.1016/S0140-6736(07)60319-5

Rose, N. (2007b). *The politics of life itself: Biomedicine, power and subjectivity in the twenty-first century.* Princeton University Press.

Schwartz, J. L. (2012). The first rotavirus vaccine and the politics of acceptable risk. *The Milbank Quarterly, 90*(2), 278–310. https://doi.org/10.1111/j.1468-0009.2012.00664.x

Sismondo, S. (2004). *An introduction to science and technology studies.* Blackwell.

Strauss, S. (2014). Ebola research fueled by bioterrorism threat. *Canadian Medical Association. Journal, 186*(16), 1206. https://doi.org/10.1503/cmaj.109-4910

Suryadevara, M., Handel, A., Bonville, C. A., Cibula, D. A., & Domachowske, J. B. (2015). Pediatric provider vaccine hesitancy: An under-recognized obstacle to immunizing children. *Vaccine, 33*(48), 6629–6634.

Weijer, C. (2020) *Explainer: How clinical trials test COVID-19 vaccines.* https://theconversation.com/explainer-how-clinical-trials-test-covid-19-vaccines-146061

WHO (2022). *WHO releases first data on global vaccine market since COVID-19.* https://www.who.int/news/item/09-11-2022-who-releases-first-data-on-global-vaccine-market-since-covid-19

CHAPTER 4

From Curated Co-Production and into the Wild West: Mass and Social Media in the Immunisation Social Order

Abstract Matters of health and medicine are commonly represented in the pages and screentime of mass news media and are hotly discussed in the realm of social media. As an intervention encouraged by the institutions that underlie the immunisation social order, and as an intervention that regularly draws controversy and dispute, vaccines are well-represented in medical coverage on both mass media and social media. Understanding how vaccines become social objects through the cultural representations created for the purposes of mass media exposition and through the dialogic and engagement-driven worlds of social media can inform our understanding of how aspects of the immunisation social order are perceived and culturally (re)shaped through various media. We uniquely centre the practices and platforms of traditional and social media within the maintenance of the immunisation social order rather than in relation to the consequences of media coverage or social media use relating to vaccine hesitancy, refusal or resistance. This chapter begins to unpack these elements first by examining through the conceptual lens of biomediatisation how we come to know and understand vaccines through mass media and how journalistic practices reshape and safeguard the immunisation social order. Following this, the role of social media and the growing field of social media analytics for the maintenance of the immunisation social order are examined, with attention given to the new possibilities that social media provides for social research and some of the challenges and limitations that are yet to be overcome in the field.

© The Author(s), under exclusive license to Springer Nature Switzerland AG 2024
T. Douglass and A. Anderson, *Vaccines in Society*,
https://doi.org/10.1007/978-3-031-61269-5_4

47

Keywords Social Media · Mass Media · Cultural Representation ·
Biomediatisation · Research Methods · Data collection

4.1   INTRODUCTION

Matters of health and medicine are commonly represented in the pages
and screentime of mass news media and are hotly discussed in the realm
of social media. As an intervention encouraged by the institutions that
underlie the immunisation social order, and as an intervention that regularly draws controversy and dispute, vaccines are well-represented in
medical coverage on both mass media and social media. Understanding
how vaccines become social objects through the cultural representations created for the purposes of mass media exposition and through
the dialogic and engagement-driven worlds of social media can inform
our understanding of how aspects of the immunisation social order are
perceived and culturally (re)shaped through various medias. We uniquely
centre the practices and platforms of traditional and social media within
the maintenance of the immunisation social order rather than in relation
to the consequences of media coverage or social media use relating to
vaccine hesitancy, refusal or resistance.

This chapter begins to unpack these elements first by examining
through the conceptual lens of biomediatisation how we come to know
and understand vaccines through mass media and how journalistic practices reshape and safeguard the immunisation social order. Following this,
the role of social media and the growing field of social media analytics for
the maintenance of the immunisation social order is examined, with attention given to the new possibilities that social media provides for social
research and some of the challenges and limitations that are yet to be
overcome in the field.

4.2   THE BIOMEDIATISATION OF VACCINES

Media portrayals of medical matters are widespread and are one of the
most common subjects in news media reporting (Briggs & Hallin, 2016).
Throughout our lives media portrayals are an important resource that
people draw on when attempting to make sense of matters of health

and illness. Though people increasingly access health information online, traditional media still play an important role; research shows that almost half of the UK population used newspapers or magazines as a source of health information when asked in 2018 and 38% in 2020 (Wellcome Monitor, 2020, 2021). However, media representations are not simply neutral disseminations of facts; portrayals of medical matters are influenced by a great many social and political factors (see Seale, 2004). Importantly, not only are images and ideas of medical objects and subjects reflected in and accompanied by media depictions, but they are also partly (re)produced and (re)created by media portrayals (Clarke et al., 2021). In this sense, notions of health, disease, diagnosis, treatment are intimately connected to, and are inseparable from social and cultural representations. In other words, they are co-produced.

The co-production (Jasanoff, 2004)[1] of health-related news coverage and the medical subjects and objects reported is central to Briggs and Hallin's (2016) notion of biomediatisation (Briggs & Hallin, 2016). Briggs and Hallin argue the relations between biomedicine and media/journalism are less distant than one might immediately think; rather biomedical subjects and objects and our understanding of them are co-produced along a boundary involving both biomedical professionals and journalists/media professionals. Understanding biomediatisation necessarily involves understanding the related processes of mediatisation and biomedicalisation, concepts which respectively refer to sets of transformations that have made both media and biomedicine central to social life (see Briggs & Hallin, 2016; Clarke et al., 2003). The concept of biomediatisation facilitates understanding of the entanglements between biomedicine and media and the influence of each sector on the other.

In this sense, vaccines and how we understand them are co-produced at the boundary between biomedicine and media. Like other medical matters, vaccines and vaccine narratives are portrayed and reproduced in media representations, and this reshapes and influences how we know vaccines. The process of biomediatisation therefore can also influence the

---

[1] Jasanoff (2004, pp. 2–3) defines co-production as "shorthand for the proposition that the ways in which we know and represent the world (both nature and society) are inseparable from the ways in which we choose to live in it. Knowledge and its material embodiments are at once products of social work and constitutive of forms of social life; society cannot function without knowledge any more than knowledge can exist without appropriate social supports".

nature, composition and maintenance of the immunisation social order. We turn now to examine some examples from the recent history of vaccines that illustrate the role played by media in (re)producing and (re)shaping how society comes to know and understands vaccines.

Drawing on interview data, research has explored the dilemmas and challenges faced by Australian journalists that relate to the portrayal of vaccines during the 2009 Swine Flu pandemic (Holland & Blood, 2012). The narratives of journalists regarding their own work help us to understand the role of this profession and how subsequent media representations of vaccines can shape how we come to socially understand vaccines. Holland and Blood (2012) show that there were conflicting expert viewpoints relating to the safety of the swine flu vaccine. This introduced a journalistic dilemma about the relative weight given in reporting to discussion of safety risks and the biomedical experts espousing these notions when it might contradict public health advice. Journalists discussed the need to 'strike the right balance' between identifying vaccine risks and the responsibility not to dissuade people from being vaccinated; getting this balance wrong could possibly influence public perception and anger vaccine experts. Indeed, one newspaper journalist in Holland and Blood's (2012) study said the following:

> I guess I was quite concerned when I was particularly writing about the adverse reactions [to the vaccine], to make sure that I was, really struck a balance between pointing out the risks and not just completely scaring people off getting the vaccine at all, that was a big concern with me and for me.

However, journalists also reported that they felt well-equipped to distinguish between worthy viewpoints and those lacking validity. In this regard, journalists approached coverage of vaccines guided by a spectrum of respectable and legitimate opinion (which partially reflects dominant biomedical understandings). At one end of this spectrum are vaccine-critical and conspiracy views and at the other are viewpoints mirroring government-issued public health advice, and journalists stated that it may be reasonable to portray legitimate expert viewpoints that differ from government advice about vaccines. For example, in a Guardian column on 'parents and parenting' in 2019, parents who are sceptical about vaccination are described as "otherwise reasonable [...] who balk at flat earthers or 9/11 truthers [but] have somehow bought into scare stories about vaccines' harmful metal content or links to disease" (O'Reilly, 2019). More recently an online article in the Telegraphy titled *"Health Secretary urged to release data that 'may link Covid vaccine to excess deaths'"* references a group of MPs trying to 'sound alarm' about "growing public and professional concerns at the UK's rate of excess deaths since 2020" and "demanding to be shown the underlying data to support the Government's assertion that there is 'no evidence' linking excess deaths to the vaccines for Covid-19" (Turner, 2024). In the comments section of the article, responses make reference to Government regulators being funded by industry, 'untested' or 'experimental gene therapy jabs' and compare the modelling of excess mortality by the Office for National Statistics with 'the global warming idiocy'. These examples illustrate how journalists use language to variously minimise or give voice to concerns around vaccines and vaccination.

Reflecting what Briggs and Hallin (2010) call a public sphere model of biocommunicability where the audience is viewed being composed of active and engaged citizens rather than patients or consumers and that a range of possibly conflicting voices will be heard, it is not in the interests of informed public debate to ignore legitimate concerns about vaccines even if this might harm or restrict the functioning of the immunisation social order. In the case of the swine flu vaccine roll out in Australia, this included disagreement about the scope and speed of the vaccination programme and the safety of multi-dose vials (Holland et al., 2014, p. 59), providing representation for debates that the public might otherwise have not been aware of. In this regard, journalistic reflexivity—relating to considerations of professional responsibility, of the impact of media coverage, as well as what represents a 'legitimate' viewpoint—is an important concept within in the co-production of vaccine narratives and understandings. These practices thus help shape how vaccines and their nature are understood within the immunisation social order and, in this regard, can frame and amplify opinion which challenges or is critical of the immunisation social order if it originated from respectable sources.

In our discussions about the history of vaccines in Chapter 2, we noted that when vaccine controversy is discussed in the public realm, the MMR-autism connection and the story of the retracted work of Andrew Wakefield often centrally feature. We noted that the continued focus on the story of Wakefield and the MMR controversy in public discourse reflects the socially productive nature of the story; the dominant narrative of the story affirming the benefits and safety of vaccination as well as the importance of trust in vaccines, health authorities and consensus science. This illustrates how, media portrayals of vaccines are important in the reproduction of the dominant narratives surrounding vaccines broadly and the MMR controversy specifically. As Conis (2017, pp. 301–302) states, the narrative has been invoked at the time of several outbreaks of vaccine-preventable infectious diseases:

> When a 2015 US measles outbreak was traced to California's Disneyland, Forbes blamed it on parents who espoused anti-vaccinationism because of Wakefield's theory. Newsweek reported similarly when measles broke out in Berlin in that same year. After Wakefield published his study, reported National Geographic, 'vaccination rates dropped in Britain and Western Europe, and [his] theory lived on in Internet chat rooms and among believers of the anti-vax movement.' The theory was behind rising rates of measles in England and Wales in 2009 and a 2008 outbreak of the disease in San Diego, reported the Los Angeles Times.

Here we see how the illegitimate end of the spectrum of legitimate vaccine opinion is discussed; for responsible, credible journalists, it must never be positively or uncritically portrayed in news media coverage. In reproducing the dominant narrative, journalists exclude, dismiss or demonise Wakefield and the worldview of his followers and thus depict Wakefield as lacking scientific credibility, as a threat to life and the central cause of considerable unfounded fear (Conis, 2017). In doing so journalists and media professionals play a role that affirms the benefits and safety of vaccines and the importance of trust in vaccines and health authorities in the co-production of the nature of vaccines and how we understand them.

The MMR-autism narrative was again central to news coverage in 2016 of the decision by the Tribeca Film Festival (later reversed) to screen a film directed by Wakefield entitled *Vaxxed*. The film focuses on a CDC whistleblower alleging that the link between vaccines and autism has been kept hidden. Journalists criticised the content of the film and argued against its inclusion in the festival (Conis, 2017) as its content lay at the wrong end of the spectrum of legitimate vaccine opinion and it would have led to greater exposure for Wakefield's ideas and thus possibly threatened the maintenance of the immunisation social order. In this sense, though journalists reflect and reproduce the biomedical consensus they also use their own social position and influence to challenge or constrain the spread of illegitimate vaccine views thus influencing how we come to know vaccines—and in the process work to preserve the immunisation social order.

4.3 SOCIAL MEDIA AND THE IMMUNISATION SOCIAL ORDER: NEW FRONTIERS AND NOVEL RESEARCH METHODS

4.3.1 *Social Media and the Changing Landscape of Vaccines in Society*

While curated mass media representations of medical technologies like vaccine continue to play a significant role in generating consensus in the cultural milieu that they are an intimate part of, social media has rapidly become a key space for understanding the state of the social practices involved in maintaining the immunisation social order. The public has increasing independence regarding health decisions, particularly in cases where vaccines are not mandatory, and combined with increased rates of online health information-seeking this has generated an international "environment where collective knowledge coexists with harmful misinformation" (Bari et al., 2022; Karafillakis et al., 2021; Malova, 2021, p. 347). Moreover, social media are not simply spaces where various kinds of information are passively posted and received. Social media spaces are interactive by their very nature, with users forming connections that become complex social network structures that reflect the pattern of information flows supported by algorithms that maximise user engagement by prioritising content that individual users are most likely to engage with and spread.

The interactive nature of social media sits alongside the growth of well-connected opposition to the institutions, laws and social practices that make up the immunisation social order—an opposition that understands how to effectively utilise the unique features of social media interactivity. Recent studies have illustrated, for example, that social media accounts from anti-vaccine communities are both highly active and are also effective at generating densely connected communities producing highly frequent and spreadable content characterized as an 'infodemic' (Hernandez et al., 2021, p. 2963; Hou et al., 2021; Hoffman et al., 2021). Behaviours used to generate this outsized influence reported in research include the production of hourly anti-vaccine content that drives traffic to these densely connected social networks (Hernandez et al., 2021), and the co-option of pro-vaccine campaigns through the hijacking of hashtags which may have been deployed following outdated guidance from medical institutions that has not kept up with the tactics of their opposition (Hoffman et al., 2021). Research has shown that negative content has a higher potential to be self-reinforcing as anti-vaccine content tends to engender more engagement which raises the probability of that content being spread to other users (Puri et al., 2020). In contrast, groups and individuals who may be broadly considered supportive of the immunisation social order, such as healthcare organisations and healthcare professionals themselves, tend to be less active or strategically aware regarding social media when it comes to the support of the immunisation social order.

4.3.2   Social Media as a Frontier for Social Research

The use of social media for social research into topics like vaccination holds significant potential for understanding the functioning and health of the immunisation social order, but there remain several challenges to be overcome ethically and methodologically. One of the key advantages of social media as a source of data compared to other data collection methods like surveys or interviews is that the scale of data collection is often orders of magnitude larger. For example, in Hou et al's (2021) 'global social listening study' the researchers collected 12,886 tweets or Weibo posts in a two-month period, Zhang et al's (2021) 'infoveillance' study analysed 156,223 social media messages, Pedersen et al. (2020) estimated that a social media campaign they evaluated reached over 8,000,000 people with an average of 127 comments per social media post from May 2017 to January 2019, Tang et al. (2021) analysed 3,731 posts on the Facebook and Twitter accounts of Canadian news organisations, and Piedrahita-Valdés et al. (2021) analysed almost 1.5 million vaccine-related tweets published between 1st June 2011 and 30th April 2019. These vast numbers of social media posts provide not only large qualitative datasets but may also contain metadata covering the characteristics of the poster, provide longitudinal attitude data for posters and include geo-locating data that can allow for local targeting. In some studies, social media data has also been connected to 'real-world' vaccination behaviour, such as in a study by Bar-Lev et al. (2021) which combined parents' social media posts and responses on Facebook and Tapuz with the vaccination records of children insured in Maccabi's Health Maintenance Organization, finding that the inclusion of social media activity data into some vaccination prediction models improved their performance. A second significant quality of social media data is that the qualitative reflections contained in the data are unsolicited rather than responsive, and therefore provide a relatively natural archive of sentiment regarding contemporary events such as health crises or changes in vaccination policy.

The quantity of available data and the speed with which new data is generated have driven the use of new methods and tools for analysis. Machine learning tools and automated or semi-automated sentiment analyses are popular; however, the field of social media monitoring is fairly new, and the evolution of analytic capacities is rapidly evolving. A challenge that arises from this is that the field lacks a "coherent body of agreed-upon methodologies", with researchers using "an amalgamation of methodological choices that sets no standards" for researching different platforms, appropriate time periods, sample sizes or the study of extreme positive or negative views that are not representative of general populations (Karafillakis et al., 2021, p. 7). Support for researchers from popular social media platforms also tends to be lacking for non-English-speaking researchers or is concentrated in certain institutions, prompting concerns evidenced by systematic reviews that much of the social media research examining, for example, misinformation has its origins in the Global North with a severe lack of insight able to be generated from the Global South (Linden, 2023, p. 1007). For our purposes, an ongoing challenge in terms of using social media analyses to understand the changing state of the immunisation social order is that insights from these kinds of data and analytics may be biased firstly towards heavier social media users who are distinct from the general population they live within based on age, gender, education and socioeconomic status, and secondly towards 'WEIRD' populations: those that are Western, Educated, Industrialised, Rich and Democratic (Henrich et al., 2010). The replication of findings across cultural and international borders to build the required knowledge base that institutions associated with the immunisation social order can use to engage with social media in the future will therefore require significant introspection from researchers engaging in social media monitoring using the ever-expanding array of available tools to mine apparently limitless data sources.

Alongside these empirical methodological frontiers, the growing field of social media analytics also harbours several challenges for research ethics. There is a lack of consistency in institutional research ethical requirements regarding social media data available online as part of the public domain. There remain issues around confidentiality and anonymisation, for example, illustrated in Karafillakis et al's (2021) review of methods for social media monitoring related to vaccination by studies that included screenshots of social media users' profile data, as well as the use of data coming from minors. Social media interventions exposing people to misinformation as part of experimental procedures also pose challenges for informed consent because the delivery mechanism is often through advertisement campaigns or the placement of interventions directly into users' social media feeds (Linden, 2023). Interventions delivered via social media also harbour the potential to exacerbate disparities for which unequal access to the internet or smart phones are symptomatic, despite some promise regarding the targeting of historically marginalised communities with tailored material to address disparities (Li et al., 2022; Marcell et al., 2022). While there is evidently significant future potential for social media monitoring as part of the practice and maintenance of the immunisation social order, researchers and the institutions they operate within still have a multitude of thorny issues to untangle to ensure that this monitoring is both empirically justified and ethically sound.

4.3.3 Interventions in Social Media: Silver Bullets or Unremarkable Outcomes?

Real-time tracking of sentiment relating to vaccines and health crises is one of the central proposals of proponents of social media monitoring which may be absorbed as part of the future of the immunisation social order. One of the main areas of utility suggested by studies investigating the potential for social media monitoring has been the connection between real-world events and social media sentiment. Bari et al. (2022), for example, suggest causal connections between vaccine eligibility during the COVID-19 vaccine rollout and Twitter sentiment in US regions, with a lag of around a week between all-adult eligibility and increases in positive sentiment, followed by increases in vaccination rates. Bari et al., (2022, pe7) conclude that their study 'highlights the potential' for sentiment analysis and natural language processing of tweets "to be part of a larger big data analytics framework to connect predictive features from social media in order to understand and predict vaccination rates". Hou et al., (2021, p. 2) similarly contend that social media has become a "source of data for detecting outbreaks and understanding public attitudes and behaviours during public health emergencies", with large real-time datasets being generated every day that could be used to support health communication and promotion messaging. Bridging the gap between a well-developed and robust social media monitoring system and the institutions and practices of the immunisation social order would seem to be the next significant hurdle once the methodological and ethical kinks have been sufficiently addressed. However, an advantage of the real-time generation of social media is that it provides a unique space for evaluation research through natural experiments to inform institutional responses as crises unfold, policies change and the relationship between vaccines and society evolves across regions, cultures and demographic or social groups.

To this end, researchers have conducted experimental interventions using social media or simulated social media platforms to attempt to improve vaccine uptake. Studies such as Daley et al. (2018) experimented a social media intervention in a Colorado-based integrated healthcare organisation, enrolling parents during pregnancy. The intervention involved participation in social media with discussion-orientated features to help parents of vaccine-eligible children to discuss the topic with other parents and contribute to "the broader public discourse and help define social norms regarding the importance of vaccination for disease prevention", with Daley et al., (2018, p. 50) finding that parents who received their vaccine social media intervention were more likely to be vaccinated on time compared with parents who did not. In another example, Hoffman et al. (2021) focused on analysing a pro-vaccine social media event revolving around the hashtag '#DoctorsSpeakUp'. Hoffman et al. (2021) found that there was a "highly coordinate response of devoted anti-vaccine antagonists" sharing ready-made coordinated content in response to the hashtag which the pro-vaccine organisers struggled to overcome. These examples illustrate that while some controlled cases of social media intervention may have benefits, interventions in the 'wild' are susceptible to significant coordinated pushback from activists.

The evidence around social media interventions is mixed, with some studies reporting successes such as Daley et al. (2018) and others finding well-organised resistance responses as in Hoffman et al. (2021), including from international disinformation campaigns that have been found to correlate with declines in mean vaccination rates (Wilson & Wiysonge, 2020). A common caution is not to take social media engagement and outreach by pro-vaccine institutions as a silver bullet solution to challenges to vaccine uptake, partly due to the challenges raised above around methodological, representation, and ethical issues, but also that social media interventions may simply "not be enough to solve vaccination concerns and enable people to make positive vaccination decisions" (Li et al., 2022 p. 253) or they may receive 'unremarkable' engagement with "no reactions, no comments, no shares, relatively few views, and [being] largely ignored" (Luisi et al., 2020, p. 4573). Even where campaigns appear to receive a positive reception, they may not be significant drivers for vaccine uptake as found by Mohanty et al. (2018) in their Facebook-based intervention aimed at increasing adolescent HPV vaccination.

In short, while social media is undoubtedly a rapidly growing field of interest with regard to the maintenance of the immunisation social order, there remains a significant lack of consensus around most aspects of the field. How do researchers best engage with the ever-changing landscape of social media when researching a contentious topic like vaccination? What are the ethical norms that should be practiced? What do monitoring tools need to achieve to be of use to healthcare professionals or institutions trying to navigate a crisis for which they believe vaccines are a solution?

4.4   Conclusion

This chapter has provided a brief introduction to the fluid and ever-changing formation of cultural representations of vaccines through mass and social media centring the practices and platforms of traditional and new media regarding maintaining or challenging the immunisation social order. The chapter began by outlining the concept of biomediatisation and relatedly highlighting the role played by journalists in the co-production of understandings within the immunisation social order. We argued that journalistic practices largely help to preserve the immunisation social order by restricting the dissemination of illegitimate viewpoints, though there is also a journalistic responsibility to reframe and disseminate views that might challenge the functioning of the immunisation social order where this is in the interest of informed public debate. The chapter then progressed to consider the role of social media and the growing field of social media analytics as part of the future of the immunisation social order. In both arenas there are ongoing challenges to the immunisation social order that contribute to the shaping of institutional and social practices underpinning the social order. While in the case of mass media, there are some constant refrains used in support of dominant biomedical consensus such as the invocation of Andrew Wakefield as a scapegoat for hesitancy towards a range of other vaccines than MMR, social media presently represents a potential patch of quicksand for proponents of the immunisation social order. The engagement-orientated, interactive and difficult-to-moderate spaces of social media represent a frontier for social research practice and ethics, and likewise they represent a target for both those who wish to maintain the immunisation social order and associated vaccine uptake levels and those in opposition. How social media are utilised as data-rich tools or intervened in to achieve messaging goals by actors across the spectrum of vaccine advocacy will likely become an ever more integral part of vaccine-focused responses to infectious disease crises and the management of public health more broadly.

REFERENCES

Bari, A., Heymann, M., Cohen, R. J., Zhao, R., Szabo, L., Vasandani, S. A., Khubchandani, A., DiLorenzo, M., & Coffee, M. (2022). Exploring coronavirus disease 2019 vaccine hesitancy on twitter using sentiment analysis and natural language processing algorithms. *Clinical Infectious Diseases, 74*(3), e4–e9.

Bar-Lev, S., Reichman, S., & Barnett-Itzhaki, Z. (2021). Prediction of vaccine hesitancy based on social media traffic among Israeli parents using machine learning strategies. *Israel Journal of Health Policy Research, 10*(49).

Briggs, C. L., & Hallin, D. C. (2016). *Making health public: How news coverage is remaking media, medicine, and contemporary life.* Routledge.

Briggs, C. L., & Hallin, D. C. (2010). Health reporting as political reporting: Biocommunicability and the public sphere. *Journalism, 11*(2), 149–165. https://doi.org/10.1177/1464884909355732

Clarke, A. E., Shim, J. K., Mamo, L., Fosket, J. R., & Fishman, J. R. (2003). Biomedicalization: Technoscientific transformations of health, illness, and US biomedicine. *American Sociological Review, 161–194.* https://doi.org/10.2307/1519765

Clarke, A. E., Jeske, M., Mamo, L., & Shim, J. K. (2021) Biomedicalization revisited. In W. Cockerham (Ed.) *The Wiley Blackwell companion to medical sociology* (pp. 125–149). Wiley-Blackwell.

Conis, E. (2017). Vaccines, pesticides, and narratives of exposure and evidence. *Canadian Bulletin of Medical History, 34*(2), 297–326. https://doi.org/10.3138/cbmh.190-21122016

Daley, M. F., Narwaney, K., & J., Shoup, J. A., Wagner, N. M. & Glanz, J. M. (2018). Addressing parents' vaccine concerns: A randomized trial of a social media intervention. *American Journal of Preventive Medicine, 55*, 44–54.

Henrich Henrich, J., Heine, S. J., & Norenzayan, A. (2010). Being WEIRD: Towards a broad-based behavioural science. *Behavioural and Brain Sciences, 33*(2–3), 111–135.

Hernandez, R. G., Hagen, L., Walker, K., O'Leary, H., & Lengacher, C. (2021). The COVID-19 vaccine social media infodemic: Healthcare providers' missed dose in addressing misinformation and vaccine hesitancy. *Human Vaccines & Immunotherapeutics, 17*(9), 2962–2964.

Hoffman, B. L., Colditz, J. B., Shensa, A., Wolynn, R., Taneja, S. B., Felter, E. M., Wolynn, T., & Sidani, J. E. (2021). #DoctorsSpeakUp: Lessons learned from a pro-vaccine Twitter event. *Vaccine, 39*, 2684–2691.

Holland, K., & Blood, R. W. (2012) Exploring the concept of "Biocommunicability" through an analysis of journalists' talk about reporting the 2009 Swine Flu Pandemic. In *Australian and New Zealand Communication Association Conference, Adelaide*.

Holland, K., Sweet, M., Blood, R. W., & Fogarty, A. (2014). A legacy of the swine flu global pandemic: Journalists, expert sources, and conflicts of interest. *Journalism, 15*(1), 53–71. https://doi.org/10.1177/146488491348046

Hou, Z., Tong, Y., Du, F., Lu, L., Zhao, S., Yu, K., Piatek, S. J., Larson, H. J., & Lin, L. (2021). Assessing COVID-19 vaccine hesitancy, confidence, and public engagement: A global social listening study. *Journal of Medical Internet Research, 23*(6), e27632.

Jasanoff, S. (2004). *States of Knowledge*. Routledge.

Karafillakis, E., Martin, S., Simas, C., Olsson, K., Takaes, J., Dada, S., & Larson, H. J. (2021). Methods for social media monitoring related to vaccination: Systematic scoping review. *JMIR Public Health and Surveillance, 7*(2), e17149.

Li, L., Wood, C., & E. & Kostkova, P. (2022). Vaccine hesitancy and behaviour change theory-based social media interventions: A systematic review. *TBM, 12*, 243–272.

Linden, S., & v. d. (2023). We need a gold standard for randomised control trials studying misinformation and vaccine hesitancy on social media. *BMJ, 381*, 1007.

Luisi, M. L. R. (2020). From bad to worse: The representation of the HPV vaccine Facebook. *Vaccine, 38*, 4564–4573.

Malova, E. (2021). Understanding online conversations about COVID-19 vaccine on Twitter: Vaccine hesitancy amid the public health crisis. *Communication Research Reports, 38*(5), 346–356.

Marcell, L., Dokania, E., Navia, I., Baxter, C., Crary, I., Rutz, S., Monteverde, M. J. S., Simlai, S., Hernandez, C., Huebner, E. M., Sanchez, M., Cox, E., Stonehill, A., Koltai, K., & Waldorf, K. M. A. (2022). One Vax Two Lives: A social media campaign and research program to address COVID-19 vaccine hesitancy in pregnancy. *American Journal of Obstetrics & Gynecology, 227*(5), 685–695.e2.

Mohanty, S., Leader, A. E., Gibeau, E., & Johnson, C. (2018). Using Facebook to reach adolescents for human papillomavirus (HPV) vaccination. *Vaccine, 36,* 5955–5961.

O'Reilly, S. (2019). *I avoid giving parenting advice—except on infant vaccines.* [Online]. https://www.theguardian.com/lifeandstyle/2019/aug/11/i-avoid-giving-parenting-advice-except-on-vaccines-seamas-oreilly. Accessed 20 March 2024.

Pedersen, E. A., Loft, L. H., Jacobsen, S. U., Søborg, B., & Bigaard, J. (2020). Strategic health communication on social media: Insights from a Danish social media campaign to address HPV vaccination hesitancy. *Vaccine, 38,* 4909–4915.

Piedrahita-Valdés, H., Piedrahita-Castillo, D., Bermejo-Higuera, J., Guillem-Saiz, P., Bermejo, H., & J. R., Guillem-Saiz, J., Sicilia-Montalvo, J. A., Machío-Regidor, F. (2021). Vaccine hesitancy on social media: Sentiment analysis from June 2011 to April 2019. *Vaccines, 9,* 28.

Puri, N., Coomes, E. A., Haghbayan, H., & Gunaratne, K. (2020). Social media and vaccine hesitancy: New updates for the era of COVID-19 and globalized infectious diseases. *Human Vaccines & Immunotherapeutics, 16*(11), 2586–2593.

Seale, C. (2004). *Media and health.* Sage Publications.

Tang, L., Douglas, S., & Laila, A. (2021). Among sheeples and antivaxxers: Social media responses to COVID-19 vaccine news posted by Canadian news organizations, and recommendations to counter vaccine hesitancy. *CCDR, 47*(12), 524–533.

Turner, C. (2024). *Health secretary urged to release data that 'may link Covid vaccine to excess deaths'.* [Online]. https://www.telegraph.co.uk/news/2024/03/02/health-secretary-release-data-covid-vaccine-excess-deaths/. Accessed 20 March 2024.

Wellcome Monitor 2020 (2021). *How the British public engage with health research.* https://wellcome.org/reports/wellcome-monitor-2020-how-british-public-engage-health-research

Wilson, S. L., & Wiysonge, C. (2020). Social media and vaccine hesitancy. *BMJ Global Health, 5,* e004206.

Zhang, Z., Feng, G., Xu, J., Zhang, Y., Li, J., Huang, J., Akinwunmi, B., Zhang, C. J. P., & Ming, W.-K. (2021). The impact of public health events on covid-19 vaccine hesitancy on chinese social media: National infoveillance study. *JMIR Public Health and Surveillance, 7*(11), e32936.

CHAPTER 5

Vaccine Inequality: The Ouroboros Within the Immunisation Social Order

Abstract Health is intimately connected to a number of social and economic inequalities at a range of scales. As an intervention that mitigates the risks posed by infectious diseases, vaccines have a role to play in alleviating many inequalities, but are themselves subject to a number of factors that reduce equality of access and uptake. These issues are the focus of this chapter: what impact can vaccines have on inequalities in society, and what are some of the issues that underpin inequalities in vaccine access and uptake? We examine both the social co-benefits relating to the reduction of social inequality produced by high levels of vaccine coverage as well as the problems or challenges to the development of the immunisation social order internationally that inequalities in access and uptake represent.

Keywords Inequality · Poverty · Social Determinants of Health · Social Justice · Social Capital · International Relations

5.1 INTRODUCTION

Health is intimately connected to a number of social and economic inequalities at a range of scales. This connection is a key concern for policymakers, illustrated through numerous reports over recent decades including in the UK the Black Report originally published in 1980 (Black et al., 1992), Acheson Report (Acheson, 1998) and Marmot Review (Marmot, 2010). As an intervention that mitigates the risks posed by infectious diseases, vaccines have a role to play in alleviating many inequalities but are themselves subject to a number of factors that reduce equality of access and uptake. These issues are the focus of this chapter: what impact can vaccines have on inequalities in society, and what are some of the issues that underpin inequalities in vaccine access and uptake? We examine both the social co-benefits relating to the reduction of social inequality produced by high levels of vaccination coverage as well as the problems or challenges to the development of the immunisation social order internationally that inequalities in access and uptake represent.

Firstly, the chapter grapples with the impact of vaccines on inequality. We use the example of the cervical cancer burden to illustrate a health challenge with inequitable risk levels for which vaccination can act as a latent mechanism for social inequality reduction. Following this, the role of vaccines as a tool to enable social mobility is also highlighted. Together we use these examples to argue that vaccination is more than just a tool for disease prevention, but also functions as a mechanism for improving some areas of social injustice.

We then turn from the role of vaccines for addressing inequalities, to the inequalities that shape access and uptake of vaccination. This area is addressed in two parts, firstly looking at international inequalities in vaccine access through the recent example of the COVID-19 pandemic, and secondly by considering sub-national social inequalities in vaccine access and uptake. Together these areas illustrate how variations in access to vaccines are exploited for the purposes of economic and soft power by countries that are able to produce and regulate vaccines faster than others, with consequent compounding effects on existing inequalities. Moving beyond international-level inequalities, some of the sub-national social inequalities that can be masked by international trends and apparent progress are examined towards the end of the chapter.

5.2   IMPACT OF VACCINES ON INEQUALITY

The central benefit of vaccination may be perceived to be the prevention or mitigation of the effect of a disease on a vaccinated individual, with the secondary benefit of population protection through herd immunity if sufficient coverage is achieved. This longstanding benefit is well-recognised, for example, in the words of Plotkin and Mortimer (1988) who described the impact of vaccination on 'the health of the world's people' as 'hard to exaggerate', contending that only safe water has had a greater impact on 'mortality reduction and population growth'. Between 2021 and 2030, it is estimated that between 44 and 63.2 million deaths will be averted due to vaccination, with an average of 5.2 million averted deaths annually over this period (Carter et al., 2023). For infectious disease context, the Review on Antimicrobial Resistance estimated that in 2050, 10 million people could die from drug-resistant infections (if nothing is done to mitigate drug resistance in the meantime) up from 700,000 annually when the report was published in 2016 (Review on Antimicrobial Resistance, 2016). Health is connected to many facets of societies' ability to function, develop and progress, and freedom from the impact of disease is not something that is distributed equally across geographic, social or economic axes. Consequently, through the impact that vaccination has on the health of individuals and populations, vaccination can also be considered a tool for social justice by improving the state of other detrimental inequalities within and between countries. In this sense, the development or maturation of the immunisation social order in countries globally can foster wider societal benefits relating to the reduction of inequality.

An example of the connection between economic and social conditions and health outcomes is the distribution of the cervical cancer burden. Poverty is a root cause of the inequality of this burden, mediated through "higher risk of HPV exposure and reduced detection, follow-up, and treatment of abnormalities" (Barbaro & Brotherton, 2014, p. 422; see also Drolet et al., 2013). The complexities of detecting, treating and engaging in surveillance of cancers require significant interaction between patients and local healthcare systems, which can be a challenge due to travel distance or an inability to take time away from work or caring responsibilities, and will of course also be impacted by the state of the healthcare system itself. Individuals who have good insurance or can otherwise access private treatment will likely be accessing a better-resourced level of care than may be available from a nationally funded healthcare service. However, HPV vaccination has been found to reduce the distance between higher and lower socioeconomic groups' incidence rates for cervical cancer even where there are differences in engagement

with healthcare systems (measured, for example, by screening participation) (Malagón et al., 2015). HPV vaccination also illustrates how
vaccination can act as a latent mechanism for inequality reduction as
the disparities between groups that tend to obtain the HPV vaccination and those who tend not to—disparities that are often evident along
socioeconomic, ethnic and religious lines—are not necessarily immediately apparent in the same way that those associated with, for example,
seasonal influenza vaccination might be (Greenwood, 2014; Polonijo &
Carpiano, 2013). The disparity between vaccinated and unvaccinated
groups becomes apparent years later when cervical cancers are more
likely to develop, rather than more immediately in the seasonal incidence of influenza. Vaccination of groups that may have reduced access
to healthcare or otherwise fewer interactions with the healthcare system
can therefore mitigate inequities that exist in healthcare outcomes later in
life, in this example by reducing the risk of cervical cancer.

By reducing the burden of diseases and their complications, vaccination
can be positioned as a social justice intervention with positive effects on
social mobility and associated economic inequities. For example, children
who face a lower disease burden and are healthier demonstrate better
school attendance and educational attainment, also being less likely to
require educational support for issues like hearing loss stemming from
mumps, rubella or other infections (Ali et al., 2022; Barham & Calimeria,
2008; Bloom et al., 2012; Deogaonkar et al., 2012; Rodrigues & Plotkin,
2020). The economic impact of childhood illnesses most immediately falls
on their carers, such as their parents, and in most industrialised nations
both parents are often involved in part- or full-time work. Forgoing work
in order to care for a sick child can result in the loss of income or
barriers to progression within some employment situations, disproportionately affecting women (Rodrigues & Plotkin, 2020). In the longer
term, improvements in infant and child mortality lead to smaller family
sizes and greater concentration of familial resources per child being raised
(Andre et al., 2008). The value of vaccination here extends beyond trade-
offs in infrastructural costs against lives saved, but incorporates many
indirect benefits in the mitigation of local economic inequities, changes in
the concentration of family units and workforce productivity, all of which
contribute to economic growth. Given the international distribution of
disease burdens which vaccines could alleviate, with higher concentrations
of mortality and morbidity in developing nations and particularly disproportionately in lower-income African nations (Carter et al., 2023), the

rationale for including vaccination as part of initiatives such as the Sustainable Development Goals becomes readily apparent given these positive externalities.

In summary, to understand why inequalities in the distribution and application of vaccination as a public health intervention are so significant, it is important to understand the impact of vaccines on a range of inequalities that stem from the burden of preventable disease. When policymakers or health economists consider interventions to improve vaccine coverage in underserved regions within countries or in countries that do not have their own fully functioning vaccination infrastructure, their improvements will not only reduce the incidence of disease but will also provide long-term benefits to the sustainability of healthcare systems, economic growth, educational attainment, the empowerment of women and a range of other social and economic boons. The development and global maturation of the immunisation social order therefore not only protects people against preventable disease, but in doing so has the potential to reduce a range of social and economic inequalities.

5.3   International Inequality in Vaccine Distribution

Inequalities in the access to and uptake of vaccines represent a challenge to the development of high levels of vaccination coverage; in other words, these inequalities restrict or challenge the growth of the immunisation social order in all countries globally and reflect problems in the network of practices and relationships that produce and protect high levels of vaccination coverage nationally and internationally. During the COVID-19 pandemic, the factors that underlie the unequal international distribution of vaccines became evermore starkly apparent not only in terms of the distribution of COVID-related mortality, but also in terms of the other social and economic impacts that separated those with the capability to adapt and respond and those who were not so well-equipped. The COVID-19 pandemic presents a particularly vivid case study because of the global ubiquity of negative effects on healthcare systems, economies and social interactions highlighting the heterogeneous concentrations of financial, technical and institutional ability to respond to the pandemic through vaccine development to mitigate health and economic impacts and begin recovery. COVID-19 also exemplifies one of the significant divisions in vaccine development in that it is a disease that threatened rich Western populations, as opposed to other neglected diseases like Chagas disease, leishmaniasis, hookworm infection and schistosomiasis that predominantly affect poor populations in Global South countries (Hotez, 2021; Molehin et al., 2022). Neglected diseases such as these which predominantly affect poorer populations generally see fewer resources dedicated to their alleviation through the costly research, development and licensing processes that go into complex biological technologies like vaccines.

One of the ongoing dangers populations face from COVID-19 is the evolution and spread of variants that may be more severe, transmissible and/or immune-evasive. Unequal global coverage of COVID-19 vaccines means more concentrated emergence of variants from within under-vaccinated regions or groups. This was highlighted in a striking example of the inequalities exacerbated by the distribution of vaccines during the first years of the pandemic when higher-income nations began providing their citizens with second or even third booster vaccinations while some lower-income nations contemporaneously lacked the means to offer first doses to the majority of their populations (Oehler & Vega, 2022). The greater concentration of risk for variant emergence within the Global South where access to COVID-19 vaccinations was limited meant that not only did the health burden fall disproportionately on countries in this region, but the ongoing socioeconomic burden arising from cases, hospital admissions and deaths fell disproportionately on these countries as well (Hassan et al., 2021; Oehler & Vega, 2021; Suárez-Álvarez & López-Menéndez, 2022). Selective travel bans, Hassan et al. (2021, p. 1) contend by way of example, were "attempts to firefight the symptoms of inequality in global access to vaccine supplies" given that in the words of the Director-General of the WHO Dr Tedros Ghebreyesus in May 2021: "No one is safe until everyone is safe" (UNICEF, 2021). The distribution of vaccines—and the underlying socioeconomic mechanisms that generated this distribution—created a global context in which the pandemic and its health and socioeconomic impacts were not only likely to be more severe, but also more prolonged as countries were able to relax non-therapeutic measures such as travel bans and shelter-in-place orders at different rates. These non-medical coping strategies were litmus tests for the penetration of the immunisation social order, highlighting the spaces and places where means for achieving COVID-19 vaccine coverage had yet to be shared.

One of the key engines of global vaccine inequality is the unequal distribution of the capacity to produce vaccines. This is a key challenge to the internationalisation of the immunisation social order geared towards producing and maintaining vaccine coverage. During the COVID-19 pandemic, the countries that were quickest to have vaccine produced within their borders were those that had both the technical capacity for research and development, and the institutional capability to authorise vaccine using emergency protocols (Fonseca et al., 2022). In the US, for example, then-President Trump pressured the Food and Drug Administration (FDA) to approve a vaccine so that he could reap political gains during an electoral cycle, while there were also concerns about the speed with which the Medicines and Healthcare Products Regulatory Agency in the UK approved a COVID-19 vaccine (Fonseca et al., 2022). These rapid institutional movements reflect the concentration of technical research, development and production capacity with which some countries were able to respond to the pandemic through the intervention of vaccines. This pace was reflected in the speed at which high-income countries achieved vaccination rates of 75–80% within the first year of the distribution of vaccines against COVID-19, compared to less than 10% among low-income countries in the same time period (Pilkington et al., 2022). This inequity broadly reflects gaps in both scientific technical and regulatory institutional capacities between developed and developing nations, as well as indicating national differences in the extent of penetration of the practices that facilitate the immunisation social order.

A long-term solution to the varied speeds at which regions of the world are able to respond to crises such as COVID-19 is to expand the technical capacity of lower- and middle-income countries, fostering the spread of the immunisation social order beyond the developed world. Production and supply chain barriers are a key constraint on equitable global vaccine distribution, with the ability to produce complex biological products like vaccines largely limited to countries including the United States, European countries, India and China while most countries in Africa broadly lack manufacturing capacity (Asundi et al., 2021) even while biological products are produced through research on their populations (Rajan, 2006). The often-demanding supply chain and storage requirements of vaccines, including significant refrigeration 'cold-chain' challenges, have been used as an argument against the waiving of trade-related aspects of intellectual property rights to facilitate technology transfer because, the argument goes, this waiving would 'make no sense' (Aryeety et al., 2021, p. 23). This further raises ethical questions regarding the pharmaceutical companies that develop and provide at-scale manufacturing of vaccines based on large amounts of public funding, only to resist conditions that may facilitate a more equitable distribution of vaccines which in the case of COVID-19 would be crucial to mitigate under-vaccinated variant breeding grounds (Hassan et al., 2021).

Given the structural barriers outlined above, the distribution of vaccines during the global crisis stage of the COVID-19 pandemic involved significant geopolitical jockeying, with the inequity of vaccine access underpinning the use of vaccines as 'diplomatic bargaining chips' (Pannu & Barry, 2021, p. e744). Vaccine development and delivery schemes were often pursued "narrowly in the name of national interest, national-state security and with a view to an economic return on vaccine development investments in pharmaceutical firms chosen as national champions" (Sparke & Levy, 2022, p. 89). Russia and China, for example, did not participate in COVAX[1] and provided their domestic vaccine candidates Sputnik, Sinopharm and Sinovac through bilateral agreements with other countries with the aim of improving their international relationships, global standing and generating strategic influence (Asundi et al., 2021). China, needing to mitigate its association with the origins of COVID-19 in its Wuhan province, made its vaccines available outside the COVAX initiative to countries left behind by vaccine inequity to displace negative sentiments with positive ones (Lee, 2023). COVID-19 additionally coincided with a rise in competition between nations and the growth of nationalist sentiments around the world such as President Trump's 'America First' stance and the UK's 'Brexit' movement underpinning the attachment of nationalist sentiment to COVID-19 vaccines, for example, as a 'Brexit Dividend' in the UK (Caliendo, 2022). Vaccines have long been used as a lever of soft power, stretching back to relations between the White House and Native American diplomats in the early 1800s (Pannu & Barry, 2021), through the Cold War, and now contemporaneously evolving through modern crises as both strategic pressures

---

[1] COVAX was an initiative jointly administered by the WHO, Gavi, the Vaccine Alliance and the Coalition for Epidemic Preparedness Innovations between April 2020 and December 2023. The initiative aimed to procure-to-donate sufficient vaccines for 92 low-income countries to vaccinate around 30% of their populations against COVID-19 (Loft, 2022).

against Western influence and as Western reinforcement of Intellectual Property and profit protection.

A corollary of having earliest access to the new COVID-19 vaccines was the ability of HICs to stockpile vaccines. As noted, for these countries, this enabled the vaccination of their populations with second and even third booster doses before some countries had managed to distribute first doses to their most vulnerable people (Rackimuthu et al., 2022). This early access and ability to stockpile was baked into agreements between governments and the pharmaceutical companies to whom public financial support was provided, for example, support from 'Operation Warp Speed' to vaccine candidates in America was conditional on priority access for US-manufactured doses, while other wealthy nations hedged their bets with agreements for initial quantities of doses from a range of pharmaceutical companies (Oehler & Vega, 2021). This behaviour, reflecting the heightened national-security approach towards vaccination as a technical solution to the pandemic, has resulted in the compounding of inequalities outlined through the areas presented above, and highlighted the need for long-term solutions to sustain the immunisation social order and avoid the "cycle of panic and neglect that generally follows emerging infectious disease threats" (Asundi et al., 2021, p. 1039).

5.4   Social Inequalities in Vaccination

A focus on unequal vaccine distribution at the international level is useful for highlighting some fundamental macro factors that inhibit access to vaccines across different regions and countries. However, the international focus can mask a range of important inequalities below the national scale which national and local healthcare policymakers wrestle with to maximise uptake in their communities. National estimates of vaccine coverage may show a promising trend, for example, but mask subnational pockets of low coverage between urban and rural areas, or indeed between affluent and deprived urban areas (Ali et al., 2022; Mosser et al., 2019; Restrepo-Méndez et al., 2016). Other inequalities that challenge or restrict the effective functioning can include measurable factors like socioeconomic gradients expressed through direct measurements such as neighbourhood deprivation indices or household incomes, but they can also be more conceptual such as expressions of social capital that exemplify the mechanics of socioeconomic impacts upon vaccine uptake or provide other explanations for variation. Measurement of relevant inequalities, and understanding their mechanics with regard to vaccine uptake, is both a persistent and important challenge because policies targeted to granular administrative geographies require reliable data to understand the extent and context of vaccine coverage problems—and thus the extent of the problems or challenges to the reproduction of the immunisation social order.

When measuring inequalities in vaccination uptake, decisions need to be made about the kinds of vaccines to focus on and relevant measures of socioeconomic and other characteristics used to explain variation in uptake. The DTP3 vaccination, for example, is useful representation of the success of the immunisation social order, because DTP3 coverage measures a country's capacity to identify and deliver three doses of vaccine to a child at pre-specified times through routine healthcare systems, thereby presenting an image of the extent to which sustainable long-term vaccine delivery is integrated into the regular activity of the healthcare system (Hosseinpoor et al., 2016). This is in contrast to a vaccination like HPV which may have lower uptake due to religious or moral anxieties associated with adolescent sexual behaviour that extends from public concern into public health behaviour including from healthcare professionals (Quinn et al., 2012; Suryadevara et al., 2015). COVID-19 vaccinations also present a specific kind of comparison, with vaccination rates rooted in a variety of emergency-related international inequalities as discussed in the previous section. Deciding which social determinants of health (WHO Commission on Social Determinants of Health, 2008) are relevant to vaccination is challenging and complex, as such determinants could include the accessibility of healthcare, quality of education and especially maternal education, the quality of homes, conditions of work and so on. In the context of vaccination uptake, common areas of focus have been along the axes of wealth which are relevant for the material aspects of living conditions, multidimensional poverty which is important for highlighting a range of simultaneous disadvantages covering areas such as health, education and living standards covered in household surveys, maternal education associated, for example, with knowledge of medical practices, social status and autonomous decision-making, places of residence relevant for proximity to services and the quality of those services, and child's sex which is relevant due to ongoing differences between child health outcomes (Arsenault et al., 2013).

In another example of inequality restricting the functioning of the immunisation social order, a common relationship between socioeconomic context and vaccination uptake is that people living in more economically deprived contexts tend to be less likely to participate in vaccination programmes (Boyce & Holmes, 2012; Crocker-Buque et al., 2017; Glatman-Freedman & Nichols, 2012; Kumar & Whynes, 2011). However, inequalities in vaccine coverage within countries do not have static relationships with the variations in socioeconomic conditions that may exist. In England, for example, Cookson et al. (2016) document that during the 1990s coverage of the MMR vaccine was lower in the most deprived quintile of neighbourhoods compared to the least deprived quintile, but this inequality reversed in the mid-2000s following the adverse press coverage precipitated by Andrew Wakefield's now-debunked connecting of the MMR vaccination with the development of autism symptoms in children. Similarly, there was socioeconomic inequality in uptake present during the pilots of the HPV vaccination in 2007–2008 which generally disappeared during the national rollout. In Canada, Drolet et al. (2013) demonstrated that inequalities in HPV vaccine uptake persisted at a reduced level after the implementation of a public vaccination programme, and that these inequalities were particularly pronounced among aboriginal ethnic groups and women immigrating to Canada who were too old to be vaccinated by school-based public programmes. Drolet et al. (2013) highlighted that women from lower socioeconomic backgrounds and aboriginal ethnicities were generally at higher risk of cervical cancer in part due to lower participation in preventive public health activities like screening. Similar socioeconomic patterns have been found in other countries like the US, Australia and the Netherlands with correlations between cancer rates, screening participation and vaccine uptake (Bach, 2010; Barbaro & Brotherton, 2014; Rondy et al., 2010). While there may be relationships between local socioeconomic contexts and vaccine uptake, these are not static relationships and instead may indicate mediations of a range of other factors like different media consumption and reaction in the case of MMR, or go hand in hand with a range of other relevant health behaviours in the case of HPV vaccine uptake. Together these highlight that, socially, maintenance of the immunisation social order presents a 'wicked' problem, lacking definitive formulation or a specific solution due to the complex interconnection of social forces that influence the uptake of vaccines.

An economic constraint that affects many areas of healthcare access is the requirement for health insurance. While some countries such as the UK have publicly funded health services that are free at the point of use and deliver services including routine vaccinations, in some countries vaccine programmes may not be fully publicly funded or the perception of a financial requirement may be discouraging even where the vaccination programme is publicly funded in an otherwise privately dominated healthcare landscape. For example, in the US the Vaccines for Children programme provides free access to the HPV vaccine for uninsured children but the cost remains a perceived barrier (Fisher et al., 2013). In Ireland, Doherty et al. (2014) found that despite infant vaccination being free, there remains inequality in which families that have private health insurance are more likely to access infant vaccinations than those without insurance. During the rollout of COVID-19 vaccines in the USA, Dirago et al. (2022) found that despite the COVID-19 vaccine also being accessible free of charge, there was a consistent association between lack of health insurance coverage and a lower likelihood of obtaining the vaccination. For the authors of the study, this finding presented the greatest puzzlement as it was not directly connected to impedance of access like factors such as a lack of internet access to hear about or book local vaccination appointments, an inability to take time off of work, concern over missing work due to side effects or being unable to obtain transportation to receive the vaccine. The authors hypothesised that health insurance captures unobserved mechanisms such as unfamiliarity with the medical system, incomplete or inaccurate information about the medical system, as well as employment circumstances. In all of these examples, actual disparities in access to healthcare signified by a lack of health insurance also indirectly correlate with lower vaccine uptake, despite access being free.

The concept of 'social capital' can help further illuminate some of the local inequality that exists in vaccine uptake. Social capital can broadly be defined contemporarily as "the idea that access to and participation in groups can benefit individuals and communities" (Gidwani, 2009, p. 689). Social capital is not something that can be purposively manufactured in a short time span; it coheres after a long history of interaction and is always anchored to places and communities, consequently containing potentially coercive elements of social surveillance and pressure to conform backed by threats of social exclusion (Gidwani, 2009). In Japan, Nagaoka et al. (2012) illustrate that at the municipal level higher levels of social capital were associated with higher vaccination rates, and suggest that this may be due to higher levels of trust in doctors, information sharing about the benefits of vaccines and an aversion to diversion from cultural norms around vaccination. Across low- and middle-income countries, Hajizadeh (2018) also hypothesises a connection between higher levels of parental education which tends to associate with higher social capital, and a higher concentration of immunisation rates among children from wealthier households. In this example, Hajizadeh (2018) contends that better-educated mothers in particular are more likely to be receptive to public health messaging relating to immunisation and may be better positioned to have good communication with healthcare professionals, hypotheses supported by other studies (Arsenault et al., 2013; Ikilezi et al., 2020). Through concepts like social capital, we can understand the process of vaccination as inherently relational, requiring trust from patients and parents, and understanding from healthcare professionals. Moreover, we can show how inequalities illustrated by more abstract relational social characteristics than gender, income and ethnicity can be associated with unequal vaccination uptake within the immunisation social order.

5.5 Conclusion

In this chapter we have introduced some of the complexity that characterises relationships between vaccination and the plethora of social and economic inequalities that exist at multiple scales in the world. The chapter opened with a discussion of the impact of vaccination on social inequalities, highlighting that via the primary goal of vaccination to reduce the incidence of mortality and morbidity from disease, vaccination can also mitigate social inequalities. Examples of these inequalities include improving educational attainment, empowering women, improving the sustainability of healthcare systems and facilitating economic growth. The COVID-19 pandemic was used as a case study to highlight some of the issues underpinning international inequalities in vaccination uptake. This exemplified some of the factors presented in the first section, for example, countries with faster vaccination not only reducing their burden of mortality but also recovering faster economically as well. The role of institutions was also highlighted as an area underpinning inequality in vaccination access between countries, alongside the benefits to economic and soft power that the role of vaccine producer brings. Finally, we outlined some sub-national social inequalities in vaccination uptake. The importance of understanding variations between vaccines and their uptake as part of measurement decisions was highlighted, and the role of economic constraints in affecting both real and perceived access to vaccination as part of access to healthcare more broadly. Less tangible characteristics such as a parent's social capital were also noted as being part of the tapestry of factors that can impact productive relationships between parents and healthcare systems through relational factors such as positive or negative pressure from peers and adherence to social norms, and variation in ability to communicate with and understand healthcare professionals.

Together the examples in the chapter illustrate the complexity of the tapestry of inequality which the immunisation social order is simultaneously compelled but unable to overcome. While freedom from vaccine-preventable disease is the end goal of the immunisation social order—a goal that would have radical impacts on ill health exacerbated by the inequalities presented in this chapter—the institutions and regulations that underlie the research, development, production and distribution of vaccines in their current form necessarily lead to unequal access to vaccines. The incentives for vaccine research and development by the largest pharmaceutical companies are financial rather than altruistic, leading to capitalistic allocation of resources to diseases affecting states that can afford large supply contracts. Vaccines can become wrapped up in grand geopolitical manoeuvres and soft power plays that are not designed primarily to benefit those with great vaccine need and poor vaccine access. Meanwhile at local levels the dynamics of healthcare system use, societal trust and cultural norms inform the social practices that produce vaccine coverage levels—whether high or low. There are many proponents and critics of the vaccine policies of the immunisation social order, however, one of the greatest challenges to the success of the immunisation social order may not be the contest between its advocates and opponents, but the very shape and functioning of its own institutions.

References

Acheson, D. (1998). *Independent inquiry into inequalities in health* [Online]. https://www.gov.uk/government/publications/independent-inquiry-into-inequalities-in-health-report. Accessed 20 March 2024.

Ali, H. H., Hartner, A.-M., Echeverria-Londono, S., Roth, J., Li, X., Abbas, K., Portnoy, A., Vynnycky, E., Woodruff, K., Ferguson, N. M., Toor, J., & Gaythorpe, K. A. M. (2022). Vaccine equity in low and middle income countries: A systematic review and meta-analysis. *International Journal for Equity in Health, 21,* 82.

Andre, F. E., Bock, H. L., Clemens, J., Datta, S. K., John, T. J., Lee, B. W., Lolekha, S., Peltola, H., Ruff, T. A., Santosham, M., & Schmitt, H. J. (2008). Vaccination greatly reduces disease, disability, death and inequity worldwide. *Bulletin of the World Health Organization, 86,* 140–146.

Arsenault, C., Harper, S., Nandi, A., Rodríguez, J. M. M., Hansen, P. M., & Johri, M. (2013). An equity dashboard to monitor vaccination coverage. *Policy & Practice, 95,* 128–134.

Aryeety, E., Engebresten, E., Gornitzka, Å., Maassen, P., & Stølen, S. (2021). A step backwards in the fight against global vaccine inequalities. *The Lancet, 397,* 23–24.

Asundi, A., O'Leary, C., & Bhadelia, N. (2021). Global COVID-19 vaccine inequity: The scope, the impact, and the challenges. *Cell Host & Microbe, 29*(7), 1036–1039.

Bach, P. B. (2010). Gardasil: From bench, to bedside, to blunder. *Lancet, 375*(9719), 963–964.

Barbaro, B., & Brotherton, J. M. L. (2014). Assessing HPV vaccine coverage in Australia by geography and socioeconomic status: Are we protecting those most at risk? *Australian and New Zealand Journal of Public Health, 38*(5), 419–423.

Barham, T., & Calimeria, L. (2008). *Long-term effects of family planning and child health interventions on adolescent cognition: Evidence from Matlab in Bangladesh.* Univeristy of Colorado.

Black, D., Townsend, P., & Davidson, N. (1992). *Inequalities in health: The black report.* Penguin.

Bloom, D. E., Canning, D., & Shenoy, E. S. (2012). The effect of vaccination on children's physical and cognitive development in the Philippines. *Applied Economics, 44*(21), 2777–2783.

Boyce, T., & Holmes, A. (2012). Addressing health inequalities in the delivery of the human papillomavirus vaccination programme: Examining the role of the school nurse. *PLoS ONE, 7*(9), e43416.

Caliendo, G. (2022). Vaccine nationalism or 'Brexit Dividend'? Strategies of legitimation in the EU-UK post-Brexit debate on COVID-19 vaccination campaigns. *Societies, 12*(2), 37.

Carter, A., Msemburi, W., Sim, S. Y., Gaythorpe, K. A. M., Lambach, P., Lindstrand, A., & Hutubessy, R. (2023). Modeling the impact of vaccination for the immunization Agenda 2030: Deaths averted due to vaccination against 14 pathogens in 194 countries from 2021–2030. *Vaccine.*

Cookson, R., Propper, C., Asaria, M., & Raine, R. (2016). Socio-Economic inequalities in health care in England. *Fiscal Studies, 37*(3–4), 371–403.

Crocker-Buque, T., Edelstein, M., & Mounier-Jack, S. (2017). Interventions to reduce inequalities in vaccine uptake in children and adolescents aged <19 years: A systematic review. *Journal of Epidemiology and Community Health, 71*, 87–97.

Deogaonkar, R., Hutubessy, R., van der Putten, I., Evers, S., & Jit, M. (2012). Systematic review of studies evaluating the broader economic impact of vaccination in low and middle income countries. *BMC Public Health, 12*(878).

DiRago, N. V., Li, M., Tom, T., Schupmann, W., Carrillo, Y., Carey, C. M., & Gaddis, S. M. (2022). COVID-19 vaccine rollouts and the reproduction of urban spatial inequality: Disparities within large US cities in March and April 2021 by racial/ethnic and socioeconomic composition. *Journal of Urban Health, 99*, 191–207.

Doherty, E., Walsh, B., & O'Neill, C. (2014). Decomposing socioeconomic inequality in child vaccination: Results from Ireland. *Vaccine, 32*, 3438–3444.

Drolet, M., Boily, M.-C., Greenaway, C., Deeks, S. L., Blanchette, C., Laprise, J.-F., & Brisson, M. (2013). Sociodemographic inequalities in sexual activity and cervical cancer screening: Implications for the success of human papillomavirus vaccination. *Cancer Epidemiology, Biomarkers & Prevention, 22*, 641–652.

Fisher, H., Trotter, C. L., Audrey, S., MacDonald-Wallis, K., & Hickman, M. (2013). Inequalities in the uptake of human papillomavirus vaccination: A systematic review and meta-analysis. *International Journal of Epidemiology, 42*, 896–908.

Fonseca, E. M. d., Jarman, H., King, E. J., & Greer, S. J. (2022). Perspectives in the study of the political economy of COVID-19 vaccine regulation. *Regulation & Governance, 16*, 1283–1289.

Gidwani, V. (2009). Social capital. In D. Gregory, R. Johnston, G. Pratt, M. J. Watts, & S. Whatmore (Eds.), *The dictionary of human geography* (5th ed., pp. 689–690). Wiley-Blackwell.

Glatman-Freedman, A., & Nichols, K. (2012). The effect of social determinants on immunization programs. *Human Vaccines & Immunotherapies, 8*(3), 293–301.

Greenwood, B. (2014). The contribution of vaccination to global health: Past, present and future. *Philosophical Transactions of the Royal Society B, 369*, 20130433.

Hajizadeh, M. (2018). Socioeconomic inequalities in child vaccination in low/middle-income countries: What accounts for the differences? *Journal of Epidemiology and Community Health, 72*, 719–725.

Hassan, F., London, L., & Gonsalves, G. (2021). Unequal global vaccine coverage is at the heart of the current COVID-19 crisis. *BMJ, 375*, n3074.

Hosseinpoor, A. R., Bergen, N., Schlotheuber, A., Gacic-Dobo, M., Hansen, P. M., Senouci, K., Boerma, T., & Barros, A. J. (2016). State of inequality in diptheria-tetanus-pertussis immunisation coverage in low-income and middle-income countries: A multicountry study of household health surveys. *Lancet Global Health, 4*, e617–e626.

Hotez, P. J. (2021). *Preventing the next pandemic: Vaccine diplomacy in a time of anti-science*. John Hopkins University Press.

Ikilezi, G., Augusto, O. J., Sbarra, A., Sherr, K., Dieleman, J. L., & Lim, S. S. (2020). Determinants of geographical inequalities for DTP3 vaccine coverage in sub-Saharan Africa. *Vaccine, 38*, 3447–3454.

Kumar, V. M., & Whynes, D. K. (2011). Explaining variation in the uptake of HPV vaccination in England. *BMC Public Health, 11*(172), 1–7.

Lee, S. T. (2023). Vaccine diplomacy: Nation branding and China's COVID-19 soft power play. *Public Branding and Public Diplomacy, 19*, 64–78.

Loft, P. (2022). *Covax and global access to Covid-19 vaccines*. House of Commons Library. https://commonslibrary.parliament.uk/research-briefings/cbp-9240/.

Malagón, T., Drolet, M., Boily, M.-C., Laprise, J.-F., & Brisson, M. (2015). Changing inequalities in cervical cancer: Modelling the impact of vaccine uptake, vaccine herd effects, and cervical cancer screening in the post-vaccination era. *Cancer Epidemiology, Biomarkers & Prevention, 24*, 276–285.

Marmot, M. (2010). *Fair society, healthy lives: The marmot review: Strategic review of health inequalities in England post-2010*. https://www.gov.uk/research-for-development-outputs/fair-society-healthy-lives-the-marmot-review-strategic-review-of-health-inequalities-in-england-post-2010. Accessed 20 March 2024.

Molehin, A. J., McManus, D. P., & You, H. (2022). Vaccines for human schistosomiasis: Recent progress, new developments and future prospects. *International Journal of Molecular Sciences, 23*(4), 2255.

Mosser, J. F., Gagne-Maynard, W., Rao, P. C., Osgood-Zimmerman, A., Fullman, N., Graetz, N., Burstein, R., Updike, R. L., Liu, P. Y., Ray, S. E., Earl, L., Deshpande, A., Casey, D. C., Dwyer-Lindgren, L., Cromwell, E. Z., Pigott, D. M., Shearer, F. M., Larson, H. J., Weiss, D. J., ... Hay, S. I. (2019). Mapping diphtheria-pertussis-tetanus vaccine coverage in Africa, 2000–2016: A spatial and temporal modelling study. *Lancet, 393*, 1843–1855.

Nagaoka, K., Fujiwara, T., & Ito, J. (2012). Do income inequality and social capital associate with measles-containing vaccine coverage rate? *Vaccine, 30*(52), 7481–7488.

Oehler, R. L., & Vega, V. R. (2021). Conquering COVID: How global vaccine inequality risk prolonging the pandemic. *Open Forum Infectious Diseases, 8*(10), ofab443.

Oehler, R. L., & Vega, V. R. (2022). Worldwide vaccine inequality threatens to unleash the next COVID-19 variant. *International Journal of Infectious Diseases, 123*, 133–135.

Pannu, J., & Barry, M. (2021). The state inoculates: Vaccines as soft power. *Lancet Global Health, 9*(6), e744–e745.

Pilkington, V., Keestra, S. M., & Hill, A. (2022). Global COVID-19 vaccine inequity: Failures in the first year of distribution and potential solutions for the future. *Frontiers in Public Health, 10*, 821117.

Plotkin, S. A., & Mortimer, E. A. (1988). *Vaccines* (2nd ed.). W.B. Saunders.

Polonijo, A. N., & Carpiano, R. M. (2013). Social inequalities in adolescent human papillomavirus (HPV) vaccination: A test of fundamental cause theory. *Social Science & Medicine, 82*, 115–125.

Quinn, G. P., Murphy, D., Malo, T. L., Christie, J., & Vadaparampil, S. T. (2012). A national survey about human papillomavirus vaccination: What we didn't ask, but physicians wanted us to know. *Journal of Pediatric and Adolescent Gynecology, 25*, 254–258.

Rajan, K. S. (2006). *Biocapital: The constitution of postgenomic life.* Duke University Press.

Rackimuthu, S., Narain, K., Lal, A., Nawaz, F. A., Mohanan, P., Essar, M. Y., & Ashworth, H. C. (2022). Redressing COVID-19 vaccine inequity amidst booster doses: Charting a bold path for global health solidarity, together. *Globalization and Health, 18*(1), 23.

Restrepo-Méndez, M. C., Barros, A. J. D., Wong, K. L. M., Johnson, H. L., Pariyo, G., França, G. V. A., Wehrmeister, F. C., & Victoria, C. G. (2016). Inequalities in full immunization coverage: Trends in low- and middle-income countries. *Bulletin of the World Health Organization, 94*, 794–805.

The Review on Antimicrobial Resistance. (2016). *Tackling drug-resistant infections globally: Final report and recommendations* [Online]. https://amr-rev iew.org/sites/default/files/160525_Final%20paper_with%20cover.pdf

Rodrigues, C. M. C., & Plotkin, S. A. (2020). Impact of vaccines; health, economic and social perspectives. *Frontiers in Microbiology, 11*, 1526.

Rondy, M., van Lier, A., van de Kassteele, K., Rust, L., & de Melker, H. (2010). Determinants for HPV vaccine uptake in the Netherlands: A multilevel study. *Vaccine, 28*(9), 2070–2075.

Sparke, M., & Levy, O. (2022). Competing responses to global inequalities in access to COVID vaccines: Vaccine diplomacy and vaccine charity versus vaccine liberty. *Clinical Infectious Diseases, 75*(S1), S86-92.

Suárez-Álvarez, A., & López-Menéndez, A. J. (2022). Is COVID-19 vaccine inequality undermining the recovery from the COVID-19 pandemic? *Journal of Global Health, 12*, 02050.

Suryadevara, M., Handel, A., Bonville, C. A., Cibula, D. A., & Domachowske, J. B. (2015). Pediatric provider vaccine hesitancy: An under-recognized obstacle to immunizing children. *Vaccine, 33*, 6629–6634.

UNICEF. (2021). *No-one is safe until everyone is safe—Why we need a global response to COVID-19.* [Online]. https://www.unicef.org/press-releases/no-one-safe-until-everyone-safe-why-we-need-global-response-covid-19

WHO Commission on Social Determinants of Health. (2008) *Closing the gap in a generation: health equity through action on the social determinants of health—Final report of the commission on social determinants of health.* [Online]. https://iris.who.int/bitstream/handle/10665/69832/WHO_IER_CSDH_08.1_eng.pdf?sequence=1

CHAPTER 6

Technology, Agency and Experimentation: Animals and Vaccines

Abstract Animals are closely intertwined with the history and contemporary application of vaccination. The growing global attention towards zoonoses, increasing institutionalisation of One Health principles in public health and the social scientific attentiveness to non-human animals following the 'animal turn' make this an opportune moment to examine the deep social relationship between animals and vaccines. This chapter grapples with four areas of this relationship: the role of animals in the history of vaccine development, the professionalisation of veterinary medicine, the use and critique of vaccination as a 'One Health' intervention and finally the collision of societal opinion and scientific practice in animal research. Through these areas of focus we illustrate that animals have not been passive participants in the history or application of vaccination, repeatedly challenging and changing the technical and societal playing field for vaccination interventions and posing new ethical questions in an increasingly interconnected and environmentally-challenged world.

Keywords One Health · Zoonoses · Veterinary Profession · Animal Turn · Animal Research · Ethics

T. Douglass and A. Anderson, *Vaccines in Society*, https://doi.org/10.1007/978-3-031-61269-5_6

83

6.1   INTRODUCTION: WHY STUDY
ANIMALS AND VACCINATION?

Non-human animals are intimately intertwined with the medical technology of vaccination. From the first experiments with inoculation, through to the infrastructure of contemporary agriculture, animals have played a crucial role in the evolution and application of vaccination as a tool for the maintenance of human and animal health. Alongside success in human vaccination with the eradication of smallpox by 1980, the other major disease eradicated by vaccines is rinderpest: an infectious viral disease of cloven-hoofed animals such as cattle, whose eradication was announced on 25 May 2011 by the World Organisation for Animal Health (WOAH, 2011). As with the various aspects of the relationship between society and vaccines examined in this book the relationship between animals and vaccines is not static and has changed, and is continuing to change, over time.

But why should social scientists pay attention to animals, let alone in the context of vaccination? The social sciences experienced an 'animal turn' in the late twentieth century and into the twenty-first century during which animals emerged firstly as an increasingly frequent focus of study in the social sciences and humanities beyond their use as representation or metaphor, and this turn has charted a transformation of animals from mere 'objects' of study to potential subjects drawing on traditions of postmodernism and feminism and the growth of ethical movements such as veganism (Ritvo, 2007; Wolfe, 2011). Broadly speaking, this transformation entails a greater attentiveness to "the instrumental position of animals, their commodification, the institutions and technologies working on them, and the continuous violence they are exposed to in a society imbued by capitalist accumulation and growth, ecocide, and systemic exploitation of all life forms" (Pedersen, 2014). Furthermore, the role of animals as part of the public health ecosystem has been increasingly acknowledged institutionally through the adoption of 'One Health' approaches to health challenges that intersect human, animal and environmental health. Craddock and Hinchliffe (2015) contend that the 'One world, one health' integrated response to shared interspecies health concerns has found its time in part due to the emergence and re-emergence of infectious diseases involving multiple hosts and vectors for which greater interdisciplinary cooperation and coordination is required. In summary, there is a confluence of both social scientific interest in animals as valued subjects of research concerning their place and role within the social, political and economic dynamics that at this point in history seem to bind all living things together in exploitative ways, and a need to address complex and interrelated health challenges that entangle humans with animals and their common ecosystems. As this chapter will lay out, vaccines play an important role in both sides of this confluence highlighting the role of animals as active agents in the shaping of vaccine histories and innovations as well as intervening in ethical challenges associated with economic growth and exploitation, taking up a multi-faceted position within the workings of the immunisation social order.

In this chapter we first examine the role of animals in the development of vaccines, and the use of vaccines to mitigate the ever-growing threat of epizootics. This examination is framed using the concept of 'One Health', which has been influential for a range of public health concerns that cross the boundaries of species distinctions and enrols animals into the immunisation social order. In many ways, this concept fundamentally reflects the history of vaccination from the early days of the technology, exemplified by the role of Blossom the cow in the story of Edward Jenner's experimentation with inoculation against smallpox. Vaccines can be used to intervene in environmental reservoirs, protect economically valuable animals and directly protect humans from diseases that may be transmitted from non-human animals. However, there are scientific and economic limitations to the deployment and understanding of these interventions.

The use of vaccines in relation to non-human animals is tied to another important medical history: the professionalisation of veterinary medicine. Expertise in the treatment of animal diseases and the role of vaccines to address public health concerns have been key tools used historically by the veterinary profession to demarcate their professional territory from, for example, medical doctors and farriers. The veterinary profession continues to grapple with questions about its current and future role in society, and there is a growing field of 'veterinary humanities' that aims to improve our understanding of the relationship between historic, contemporary and future challenges associated with veterinary medicine, the professionals who practice it, and the expertise that they can bring to bear. We provide a small contribution to this field by highlighting the place of vaccination within veterinary history and contextualising this position with the broader One Health and immunisation social order contexts.

6.2   ANIMALS' AGENCY
AND THE HISTORY OF VACCINATION

The agency of animals has been of historic significance to the social development of vaccines and the technologies that enable their development, transportation and use—and, as such, the development of the immunisation social order. The broader history of vaccination has been covered in Chapter 2, and so this section will not re-cover the key historical points but rather will briefly examine some of the more specific aspects of animals' relationship with society and vaccines.

In the early days of vaccination, there were significant geographic challenges involved in the research, development and application of vaccines. One of the threatening features of smallpox was its transmissibility between humans without the need for alternative hosts among the animal population. Cowpox, the disease Jesty and then Jenner observed milkmaids and farm labourers catching and acquiring smallpox immunity from, was much harder to catch directly, and because the disease in cows was difficult to distinguish from other bovine diseases vaccinators relied on the extraction of lymph from infected humans. On top of this, "the natural occurrence of cowpox was sporadic and geographically specific" which meant that "would-be vaccinators depended on a foreign source of cowpox lymph" in order to perform the procedure in which the lymph was transferred into another human (Rusnock, 2009, p. 21). In the early years of vaccination, these sources were "generally limited to Gloucestershire, Lombardy, and London" according to Rusnock (2009, p. 22), drawing upon correspondence between European physicians and Edward Jenner. These early vaccinators innovated a range of approaches and technologies to try and reliably transport lymph through international networks often reliant on personal connections. These technologies included the use of threads, glass plates, specially modified lancets, and various kinds of insulation to develop the necessary systems for vaccination to travel around the world, and were a key focus of the efforts of early vaccinators because of the difficulty in finding infected cows and differentiating cowpox from other bovine diseases.

Animal-related challenges in the distribution of vaccines and vaccination continued beyond cowpox. Following the development of the polio vaccine, for example, Britain required a constant supply of rhesus monkeys from its colonial network to scale the production of the vaccine. This requirement spurred attention to and greater regulation by colonial authorities of the capture, sale and transport of rhesus monkeys in India which often relied on local and tribal efforts (Quick, 2023). In the nineteenth century, a rabies outbreak in South Africa necessitated the rapid sourcing of a rabbit population due to the need for rabbit spinal cords in the production of rabies vaccine and the lack of a local rabbit population. These challenges have led to further technological innovations and 'care tinkerings' in animal research supply chains which continue to this day (Peres & Roe, 2022) and serve to highlight animals' sometimes disruptive role as "supplier and standardizer of biological products for use in humans" (Woods et al., 2018, p. 256). Animals' bodies and their distribution within, and relationship to, environmental factors significantly shaped the often-haphazard nature of early vaccination, contributing significant agency to the directions pursued by vaccinators and the geographic networks developed in response to disease crises that spurred the growth of the immunisation social order.

In addition to the development of international networks of technological innovation and animal transportation, vaccination and the development of the immunisation social order was tied to the development of veterinary professionalisation. As Woods (2017, p. 496) has argued, histories of medicine tend to focus "on human healers and their human patients, while animal healers and patients are compartmentalized into the separate sphere of veterinary history" despite the performance of veterinary medicine having historically been the province of 'medical men'. The construction of 'veterinary expertise' and the specialisation and professionalisation of the medical care of animals has a storied history (see for example Bonnaud & Fortané, 2020, 2021; Gardiner, 2014; Woods, 2007; Woods & Bresalier, 2014), and vaccination plays a critical role in this history contextualised by the public health dangers of diseases like rabies and anthrax, concerns over malnutrition and 'protein crisis' (United Nations, 1968) and economic challenges in agricultural production. For example, in her study of the transformation of dairy farming between 1930 and 1950 and the increased dependence on domestic food production in the UK Woods (2007, p. 462) contends that "veterinary expertise had to be actively created and made relevant to the new context", and the leaders of the burgeoning veterinary profession secured this relevance by establishing a government-backed scheme for the control of diseases of dairy cows. There was significant language used to frame this expertise, as a government committee report referred to the veterinary practitioner as no less than the "physician of the farm and the guarantor of the nation's food supply", and the scheme "represented a deliberate attempt to win employment for the profession by making its expertise directly relevant to the war effort, and restructuring farmers' attitudes towards animal health and veterinary intervention" (Woods, 2007, pp. 474–475). Veterinarians used cutting-edge vaccination technology to control diseases like brucellosis with the aid of Government-subsidised vaccination. While war fronts opened in the Mediterranean and Far East which favoured animals over motorised transport led to the de-reserving of the veterinary profession and their co-option into the war effort abroad, the construction of veterinary expertise as crucial to the maintenance of agricultural production during the war (with the help of vaccination among other interventions) contributed to the passage of the Veterinary Surgeons Act in 1948, which banned unqualified practice in the UK, moved veterinary education into universities and perpetuated the wartime shift towards productivity-orientated agriculture by growing the capacity for veterinary research.

6.3   Vaccination and One Health

As should be readily apparent from the increasingly prevalent and visible effect of zoonotic pathogens—pathogens that can spread between non-human animals and humans and cause disease—on society, human and animal health are closely intertwined. This kind of transmission can occur in many ways: direct contact with the bodies and fluids of non-human animals such as through petting or scratches, indirect contact within non-human animals' habitats such as barns or coops, vector-borne transmission by ticks or insects, food contamination via undercooking or poor hygiene and water contamination for example by faeces of infected animals. Some infectious diseases are high-profile examples of zoonoses, such as rabies, Ebola Virus Disease and various acute respiratory syndromes such as MERS. Others are less-visible but routinely prevalent, such as salmonellosis. In response to the growth of zoonotic threats to public health, the concept of a 'One Health' approach has been increasingly adopted and institutionalised in policy and practice with application to the functioning of the immunisation social order.

'One Health', also sometimes referred to as 'One World, One Health', is a somewhat elastic concept that broadly is used to characterise public health challenges in which human, animal and environmental health are intertwined. The concept is not a neutral expression of the complexity of 'health' and 'disease', but is itself intertwined with professional, institutional and political challenges and aspirations. For example, 'One Health' has been suggested as a 'veterinary land-grab' (personal communication in Gibbs, 2014, p. 90) and it has been argued that One Health research is "dominated by veterinarians and animal health scientists" predominantly based in the global North (Galaz et al., 2015, p. 19). The 'common sense' interconnection that One Health underscores is not unproblematic, argue critiques of the concept (Hinchliffe, 2015, p. 28). One Health, Hinchliffe (2015, p. 30) contends, posits "material linkages between people, wild and domestic animals and ecosystems [which generates an] image of a single, bio-communicable planet, with WHO response structures at its centre, and with a well-known scenario once communing, or sharing of 'life', outstrips immunity". This image foregrounds transmission as a central pillar for intervention, but Hinchliffe argues that "even in the core of modernized framing practice, health is dependent on more than reduced transmission and regulatory fixes. Health is socio-economic and any health programme needs to address how disease risks are configured in particular socio-economic and cultural settings". Beyond its institutional significance as an acknowledgement of the complex interconnections between non-human animal and human health therefore, One Health also suggests attention to environmental influences on health in this sphere such as encroachment on ecosystems exemplified through deforestation and the exposure that forest workers to endemic diseases (Chomel et al., 2007; McMichael & Butler, 2007), the conditions in which farmed animals live, or the conditions in which farm workers labour (Hinchliffe, 2015), for which medical mitigations like vaccinations or antibiotics are quick fixes for other welfare challenges. All this is to note that while the immunisation social order plays an important role in the mitigation of zoonotic public health challenges, it is worth being critical of where vaccination does fit into the broader ecosystem of 'One Health' approaches to public health, how interventions are framed, and who is suggesting or implementing them.

There have been examples of vaccination interventions to address complex One Health challenges. Hendra virus is a zoonotic paramyxovirus discovered in 1994 in Australia during an outbreak involving 21 stabled racehorses and two humans (Daniel, 2023). For horses, Hendra is a serious respiratory and neurological disease which kills around 75% of infected horses. Hendra virus has been transmitted from infected equids to humans who were treating them, with seven known cases and four deaths. The four species of flying fox (*Pteropus* bats) found on mainland Australia are the most significant natural reservoir for Hendra virus (Middleton et al., 2014). During 2011 there were a series of Hendra horse infections in a 3-month period over a wide geographic range, which evidenced that the virus was an 'unmanaged emerging disease' (Middleton et al., 2014, p. 373). These incidents triggered a rise in media reports with a focus on the role and control of flying foxes encroaching on human settlement as disease carriers while minimising the role played by horses in transmitting Hendra to humans (Degeling & Kerridge, 2013). Due to the reduction in their natural habitats from human activities and urbanisation, some species of flying fox are endangered and were legally protected in some parts of Australia. The increased reliance of flying foxes on commercial orchards and urban gardens for sustenance meant that they had become a visible and apparently thriving pest in the eyes of some of the people living in close proximity to them. The 2011 Hendra outbreaks "permitted opponents of current [flying fox] policies and practices to reframe the issues, recast debate about what types of actions needed to be taken, and then prime the public as to how these actions could and should be justified in the face of imperfect scientific knowledge" (Degeling & Kerridge, 2013, p. 161). Horses were cast as victims alongside humans rather than being the intermediate host between the flying foxes and humans, and the increasingly politicised debate over what should be done to control Hendra virus were framed by opponents of flying fox protections as clashes between people at risk and scientists and environmentalists, and questions were raised about the "value orientations of those in authority" (ibid.). Thus, Hendra virus was not only a genuine public health risk that had led to the deaths of horses and humans, but it entangled broader environmental health questions associated with the crucial environmental role played by bats in pollination and insect population control, and ethical challenges regarding population control measures enacted by humans such as permitting the shooting of bats.

The eradication of flying foxes, while being a potentially obvious source of 'action' for policymakers, "would pose extraordinary operational challenges, notwithstanding attendant moral, ethical, and environmental issues" and being impractical for rural communities (Middleton et al., 2014, p. 373). The development of a vaccine for the prevention of Hendra virus disease in horses (Equivac®HeV, launched by Pfizer Animal Health in 2012) was therefore not only an intervention to protect horses, but also to break the chain of transmission of Hendra virus to humans and remove momentum towards the implementation of population control policies towards environmentally-important bat populations. The Australian Veterinary Association for example has previously framed the vaccine as providing "a work health and safety as well as a public health benefit" (Australian Veterinary Association, 2012).

Veterinarians themselves face numerous challenging decisions when confronted with unvaccinated horses that have contracted Hendra as they balance the public health need to perform prompt case recognition and prevent potentially fatal human infections with "substantial health and financial risks, [...] legislative obligations, [and] indemnity liability obligations in a context in which they have limited control of the actions of others and restricted treatment options" (Annand et al., 2020, p. 271). Many equine veterinarians in Australia have restricted their practice to only consult for vaccinated horses and potentially forfeit future income through the loss of clients, while others have left equine work or moved to practice in lower risk regions of the country to avoid the occupational risk that Hendra virus poses (Australian Veterinary Association, 2012; Mendez et al., 2012). This evidences a concrete indirect effect of the immunisation social order on the functioning of professional veterinary practice outside the central focus of disease mitigation.

The example of Hendra virus is a case study in the role vaccines can play within the One Health approach to public health and highlights the need to consider the critiques highlighted earlier in this section. While the vaccine provides direct benefit to horses by protecting them from the disease (Tan et al., 2018) without appearing to impede racehorse performance (Schemann et al., 2018), it has also played a role in maintaining protections for some environmentally-important species of flying fox and reducing risk for humans coming into contact with horses. However, flying foxes were only endangered and so reliant on human-populated areas for sustenance because of previous human activity and urbanisation, and on this issue the response by the institutions of the immunisation social order was something of a quick fix mitigating further harm to flying fox species without addressing more systematic issues affecting their populations. The story of Hendra virus, bats, horses and humans is by no means complete, and it has been suggested that cases of Hendra virus are likely to expand across Australia due to climate change (Yuen et al., 2021). This could perhaps be considered a multispecies justice externality of the usual functioning of the immunisation social order.

When considered in the context of the interconnections between human, animal and environmental health(s) under the umbrella of 'One Health', vaccination can become a thrice-valuable intervention. There are other examples of vaccination being used in One Health contexts beyond Hendra virus, such as vaccination programmes immunising wild animals against rabies using oral baits, and human and veterinary vaccines against West Nile virus disease that were developed with clinical trial data informing vaccine development shared across contexts (Monath, 2013). However, the various utilities of vaccination for the One Health paradigm in the context of the immunisation social order are not without potentially problematic issues if they mask other systemic challenges associated with environmental harms or poor agricultural regulation relating to non-human animals or human agricultural labourers, and for social scientists their use should not be considered uncritically.

6.4   ANIMAL RESEARCH AND VACCINES: WHERE SOCIETAL CONDITIONS AND PUBLIC OPINION COLLIDE

Prominent historic examples of diseases addressed by the development of vaccination were catalysts for advances in the use of animals for research that has driven forward the development of the immunisation social order, though sometimes with less-than-ethical approaches. Pasteur's laboratory work on vaccines against rabies for example received close scrutiny from anti-vivisectionists amidst fears that "cruelty to animals [would be] institutionalised" in a 'Millennium of Pasteurism' (Pemberton & Worboys, 2007, p. 105). Indeed, Pemberton and Worboys (2007, p. 106) reflect that 1884 readers of La Figaro "must have relished being told of the problems Pasteur faced trying to expand his laboratories, when local residents complained about the noise from his 'menagerie', their fears about living next to 'rabies factories', and falling property values". Nonetheless, as Jenner brought medical legitimacy to vaccination (described in Chapter 2), the work of the Institut Pasteur in Paris enrolled animals in research moving rabies "from the margins of medicine and veterinary practice to become iconic for both professions" (Pemberton & Worboys, 2007, p. 132) and providing groundwork for the control of rabies through vaccine technologies incorporated into the burgeoning immunisation social order and continued in international travel regulations today and in wildlife programmes using vaccine-laced bait as described earlier in this chapter.

Public opinion matters greatly for vaccination as a public health intervention and for the continued and effective functioning of the immunisation social order. This has been exemplified in previous chapters in the context of the history of vaccination and development and regulation. Vaccines cross-over with other areas where public opinion intersects with policy and regulation around society's relationship with non-human animals. The regulation and practice of animal research is one example influenced by 'public' opinion whether through sweeping measurement in opinion surveys or by the inclusion of 'lay' members of the public in the Animal Welfare Ethical Review Bodies (AWERBs) that are a legal requirement for UK animal research establishments (Davies et al., 2022; Gorman & Davies, 2020; Hobson-West, 2010). While vaccines are trialled and batch tested using animals in research laboratories, medical and veterinary vaccines are not regulated in the same way. For example, while the batch testing of vaccines for medical and veterinary use is covered by the Animals (Scientific Procedures) Act 1986, clinical trials of veterinary medicines required for marketing authorisations are not, instead being regulated through the Veterinary Medicines Directorate (VMD) (Palmer et al., 2021). This, Palmer et al. (2021, p. 124) argue, may relate "largely to which activities are perceived – by regulators, the general public, or interest groups – to be 'risky', and what kind of resistance is shown by researchers to further regulation". This intersection between public opinion of vaccines and animal research, and the practice of vaccine development and testing, presents a prism for our understanding of how controversial areas of scientific and medical practice interact with social opinions and norms.

The development of vaccines involves both non-human animals and humans as clinical trial participants at different stages of the development process. During the development of vaccines against COVID-19 the testing process was expedited, and when vaccines reached the stage at which they were tested in humans there was a push for volunteers to participate in trials to generate as much data as quickly as possible. During the development of the 'Oxford' vaccine, Vanderslott et al. (2021) studied the views of human vaccine trial participants regarding animal research through the lens of co-production. The authors state that their view of co-production in the context of animal research "emphasizes removing the boundary between 'the natural' of animals and science and 'the social' of political power, culture, and public views" (Vanderslott et al., 2021, p. 3). In their study, Vanderslott et al. (2021) examined how human

COVID-19 vaccine clinical trial participants' identities as test subjects were produced in relation to research animals in order to provide insight into interspecies subjectivities and identities. This kind of nuanced qualitative research into public perspectives on animal research is valuable for understanding the ever-changing relationship between society and animals and how public opinion legitimises animal research, with vaccine trials presenting a particular case study in how the risks and benefits of animal research which underpin the ongoing technical scientific innovation of the immunisation social order are evaluated.

In the study, Vanderslott et al. (2021, p. 20) found participants 'typically' articulated the idea that animal testing is a "necessary evil for developing medicines aimed at saving human lives, but still as something that made them uncomfortable, and which would be unjustified for frivolous purposes such as cosmetic production". While the views of what was a well-educated and pro-science sample were broadly reflected in current law around animal research in the UK, the authors noted that misconceptions about the (illegal) use of animals for cosmetic testing still cast a deep shadow. This perspective presents animal research as something that is not universally justifiable, but rather is dependent on the reason for the research being carried out as well as the methods and quality of the science. Participants in the study also used animal metaphors like 'guinea pig' and 'lab rat' "to express their sense of contributing to society and protecting the vulnerable during a health crisis", tying their voluntary participation with 'notions of civic responsibility' that were prevalent in popular discourses during the COVID-19 pandemic (Vanderslott et al. 2021, p. 21; see also Bourgeois et al., 2020). Participants quoted by Vanderslott et al. (2021, p. 18) referred to being a guinea pig to 'do my bit', or conversely to highlight "the risk involved because you're asking people to essentially be guinea pigs". While the volunteers who participated in the interview study saw their participation in the vaccine trials as the actions of model citizens, they distinguished between their own free choice and the coercion required for animals' participation and the animals were not considered as model citizens in the same way, if at all. One participant in the interview study did elaborate on a perspective that acknowledge solidarity with the animals used for research, articulating that they participated in the vaccine trials to put "my money where my mouth was [...] if I want to live in a world where there's no animal testing then I have to be prepared to put myself forward" (Vanderslott et al., 2021, p. 19). Despite these distinctions within the perspectives of participants, participants did view animals as the most suitable initial test subjects and found animal testing to be "reassuring, providing confidence in the safety of the vaccine" which suggests a degree of faith in the "model organism concept whereby animals are assumed to be reasonable proxies for humans" despite its known shortcomings (Davies, 2010; Vanderslott et al., 2021, p. 21). Although these participants were highly self-selecting for pro-science and pro-vaccine attitudes due to their sampling from a group of a vaccine trial participants, the perspectives that Vanderslott et al. (2021) draw out through their interviews highlight the nuance with which attitudes towards controversial topics like animal research and vaccines intertwine. While animal research is not seen as desirable, participation in the process alongside animals was seen as a form of civic duty for some and an act of solidarity for others, all the while 'doing one's part' to mitigate a global health crisis that was radically changing how society functioned. This contrasts with other forms of vaccine development such as the use of synthetic vaccines in livestock, for which lay people have been found to invoke associations between 'naturalness' and risk to voice opposition (Ditlevsen et al., 2020). These studies, which humanise the connection between animal research and vaccination, give voice to the societal milieu within which the practices of the immunisation social order must perform. Specifically, vaccines are only partially represented by the needle or tablet through which they are graphically delivered; many other institutions with their own social frontiers are enrolled in the service of the immunisation social order.

Issues of ethics in the history of animal use for vaccine research within the emerging immunisation social order are not limited to the animals themselves. British colonial authorities and veterinary services for example took advantage of asymmetric racial power relations to advance research agendas relating to vaccination in early twentieth-century South Africa. The 'avirulent' anthrax vaccine invented in 1930s and field-trialled in 1936 by Max Sterne (a veterinary scientist and bacteriologist working in South Africa in the 1930s and 1940s) greatly benefited from these societal dynamics, and this vaccine remains a key tool in the immunisation social order as the basis for contemporary animal vaccination against anthrax and for research into human vaccination (Gilfoyle, 2006). Concerns over the restriction of pastoral exports from South Africa due to anthrax contamination led South African veterinary scientists to try and technologically innovate improved vaccines. While white farms employed hygienic measures and a voluntary vaccination approach which failed to have a significant effect on levels of anthrax, in predominantly African-farmed areas like the Transkei large-scale compulsory vaccination was enforced owing to state veterinarians' "racially biased explanation of the incidence of anthrax" and the abandonment of enforced hygienic measures as 'impractical' in such areas (Gilfoyle, 2006, pp. 488–489). Not only was vaccination enforced in these areas, but veterinarians vaccinating African-owned livestock performed the procedure themselves rather than allowing the owners to perform the vaccination as they did in other areas. Not only did this policy mismatch highlight the segregationist nature of the society, but also enabled state veterinary scientists to obtain large amounts of statistical data required for the evaluation of Sterne's newly-invented vaccine as Transkei cattle were all vaccinated annually in conditions sufficiently controlled as to have the status of 'an extensive experiment' (Gilfoyle, 2006, p. 488). The societal conditions in 1930s South Africa thus enabled the testing of new vaccine technology which "subsequently achieved worldwide currency" (Gilfoyle, 2006, p. 490). This example illustrates that the immunisation social order is heavily influenced by the societal conditions in which it develops and evolves, deploying vaccination as a tool for public health mediated by colonial inferences about regions like the Transkei.

6.5   VACCINATION AND PARTICIPATION IN THE VETERINARY REGIME

Vaccination is a routine part of veterinary work. Within the current scope and organisation of the immunisation social order, companion animals are routinely vaccinated against diseases like kennel cough and distemper, and farm herds are vaccinated against a range of diseases such as orf disease in sheep and enteritis in cows among several others. Indeed, as mentioned in the opening lines of this chapter, one of the two diseases eradicated through vaccination is rinderpest in cattle. As Swabe (1999, p. 153) illustrates,

> to understand the nature of veterinary work, one must forget the popular image of the intrepid animal doctor battling to save the lives of sick and injured animals. [...] In reality, veterinarians are preoccupied with performing highly routine procedures pertaining to the management, control, and prevention of disease and parasitic infection.

Despite being highly routine, the vaccination of animals is not always a simple or isolated procedure and exists within broader contexts such as the client relationship within veterinary practice, practical husbandry knowledges within farms and themes of 'expertise' which are embedded within the routine functioning of the immunisation social order.

Vaccinations form a routine part of companion animal care, however the preventative health consultations within which vaccinations take place are often not solely focused on the vaccination itself. Robinson et al. (2015) for example found that preventative health consultations in small animal practice tend to involve the discussion of a greater number of problems than consultations for specific health problems, quantifying in their study that up to eight different problems were discussed in some preventative healthcare consultations. Robinson et al. (2022, p. 13) elaborate, "preventative healthcare consultations are far from being 'just a vaccine' or the 'quick and easy' consultations they are often perceived to be" and are no shorter than problem-based consultations (Everitt et al., 2013; Robinson et al., 2014; Shaw et al., 2008). During a typical vaccine booster consultation, veterinarians routinely perform several aspects of clinical examination including chest auscultation, abdominal palpation and visual examinations a well as discussing other topics such as neutering (Robinson et al., 2019). Expectations around the content of preventative healthcare consultations vary between veterinarians and between veterinarians and pet-owners (Belshaw et al., 2018). Some veterinary surgeons reported to Belshaw et al. (2018) that preventative healthcare consultations were a rewarding and important part of their work, while others found them not to be as stimulating as other areas of their work. Meanwhile, pet-owners in Belshaw et al.'s (2018) study often expected more than just a vaccination from the consultation and reported dissatisfaction when the consultation fell short of this.

These aspects of the preventative healthcare consultation highlight the sometimes challenging relationship between veterinarians as healthcare workers who are required to turn a profit, and pet-owners as clients expecting a return on their expenditure. The friction that the nature of this relationship can cause has been examined in depth in other studies with impacts upon the kind of care that veterinarians are able to provide and patients receive (see, e.g. Morris, 2012; Volk et al., 2011). As Robinson et al. (2022, p. 15) summarise, "preventative healthcare consultations are highly complex and represent an important opportunity to address a variety of pet health issues with animal owners [and] it is during these conversations that complex issues, such as vaccine hesitancy, can be identified and explored fully". Vaccination in companion animal care is therefore not a completely routine or context-free procedure as it is situated within a much broader primary care situation and has additional framing within a business-client relationship, highlighting challenges that might be faced in terms of trust or financing beyond 'hesitancy' itself. Further, this evidences an area in which the immunisation social order has come to function alongside and through other areas of care in which immunisation is only one intervention among several.

One useful barometer of companion animal vaccination in the UK is the 'PAW Report' produced by the PDSA, which includes a representative panel survey carried out by YouGov. The 2022 report (PDSA, 2022) noted that the current cost-of-living crisis may be having a detrimental effect on the ability of pet-owners to provide preventative healthcare for their animals, citing for example that 14% of surveyed dog owners considered regular booster vaccinations to be too expensive. This challenge was combined with the ongoing staffing challenge for veterinary practice in the UK which has been well-documented in the veterinary literature owing to issues such as poor work/life balance, difficult clients, emotional distress and a significant mental health crisis within the profession (Adam et al., 2019; Anderson & Hobson-West, 2022; Clarke et al., 2016; Hagen et al., 2020; Hatch et al., 2011; Montoya et al., 2021). The PAW report highlighted that this challenge meant that some pet-owners could not access preventative care for their animals because of a lack of capacity within the veterinary sector. Combined with the complexity and challenge of preventative healthcare consultations outlined above, further problems around access and a poor economic climate are compounding factors for ongoing efforts to maintain the high levels of vaccination coverage that the institutions of the immunisation order seek in animals as well as humans.

A number of studies have tried to gauge the factors associated with vaccine uptake and refusal with regard to companion animals, with several variations of online convenience sample surveys in different contexts noting similar trends. Across an international range of such studies, the provision of advice by veterinarians is often positively associated with the uptake of companion animal vaccinations as well as the use of animal boarding services like catteries and foreign travel with a companion animal (Eschle et al., 2020; Evason et al., 2021; Gehrig et al., 2019; Filipe et al., 2021; Habacher et al., 2010; Schwedinger et al., 2021). Expanding on the PAW Report's inferences regarding cost-of-living challenges, the perceived importance of cost when considering vaccination decisions have been associated with lower likelihood of feline vaccination uptake (Filipe et al., 2021; Habacher et al., 2010). However, despite the consistencies of some of these trends, online survey samples have consistent flaws such as the exclusion of the digitally disconnected, biasing towards more educated and computer literate respondents (Paolacci & Chandler, 2014; Woods et al., 2015). Approaches like the one used for the PAW Report mitigate this data quality issue in the UK, and there have been other attempts to improve data quality to further our understanding of companion animal vaccination and its social aspects. One example is 'SAVSNET', an almost real-time surveillance study operating at the University of Liverpool in which a convenience sample of veterinary surgeons in Great Britain record information at the end of their consultations which is then uploaded securely within 24 hours to be available for analysis (SAVSNET, 2016). One study published using SAVSNET practice data examined the use of vaccines and factors associated with variability in uptake for dogs and cats in participating practices (Sánchez-Vizcaíno et al., 2018). While the study found different levels of recorded vaccination to those reported through the pet-owner survey of the contemporaneous PAW Report, the relative distributions were the same with dogs being most likely to have received vaccinations, followed by cats and then rabbits. Living in less deprived areas and having pet insurance were both associated positively with having a recorded vaccine history, along with pedigree and neutered statuses. This illustrates that across different data types, there is a consistent narrative regarding finances as a challenge to companion vaccine uptake and thus the maintenance of this aspect of the immunisation social order, but also highlights with other studies the interlinking and complexity of uptake patterns with other practices likes boarding, neutering, pedigree preference and travel.

6.6   CONCLUSION: THE EVOLVING RELATIONSHIP BETWEEN ANIMALS AND VACCINES

This chapter began by contending that non-human animals are intimately intertwined with the medical technology of vaccination. This choice of words was deliberate, and as the chapter progressed, some of the intimacies around the sharing of microbial risk become apparent as well as a challenge to the idea that vaccines are indeed a 'medical' technology.

The trajectory of vaccine research, the ways that crises are responded to and the associated growth of the immunisation social order have been shown to be influenced by the distribution of animals from the early requirements for cowpox lymph to the need for to monkey and rabbit body parts in laboratory locations where populations of these animals were not immediately available. The environmental distributions of these animals meant that vast human networks and infrastructures were developed to supply locations where vaccine research and development was conducted with the animals required to conduct experiments and testing.

Vaccines were highlighted as one crucial component in the broader development of veterinary professionalisation, providing veterinarians with the tools to control diseases that threatened agricultural production. In the veterinary-dominated arena of 'One Health', an institutional alignment which shapes the practice of the immunisation social order in areas where close alignment between human and veterinary medicine is necessary for public health, vaccines were shown to play roles in mitigating zoonotic public health challenges as well as intervening in some environmental challenges.

Public opinion around vaccines and animals must be considered to encompass not only the vaccine technology itself and its application to human and non-human bodies in healthcare contexts, but also the role of animal research in developing and maintaining the technology. As with attitudes towards vaccination, public attitudes towards animal research are complex, nuanced and exist on a spectrum and may support or challenge the immunisation social order. These were illustrated for example using anti-vivisectionist sentiment around the Institut Pasteur and the early work on rabies vaccines, and the recent development of vaccines to address the COVID-19 pandemic. The measurement of attitudes towards animal vaccination in the veterinary sphere has been understudied relative to the human medical context, and this chapter has drawn out some consistent narratives from work carried out so far and noted some of the few higher-quality sources of information on this topic. This chapter contends that both attitudes towards animal research and the challenges involved in animal vaccination are objects of concern for proponents of the immunisation social order.

Vaccines have provided many benefits in the context of animals and society including the maintenance of food supplies and the mitigation of diseases that affect animals and diseases that are zoonotic. However, the history of animals and vaccines, and the associated development of the immunisation social order, is not solely about positive progress. As seen in some of the examples used in this chapter, agricultural vaccination policies of the immunisation social order—broadly conceived— have reflected discriminatory biases through the work of colonial state veterinary services, and they may sometimes be used to mask systemic challenges to welfare where regulation or husbandry fall short.

Looking forwards, with a growing world population and significant environmental challenges around urban encroachment and climate change, vaccines and the expansion of the immunisation social order may play an ever-greater role in the management of not only animal health, but human and environmental health as well. A concurrent challenge will be ensuring that the deployment of vaccine technology through the workings of the immunisation social order does not simply paper over the systemic issues that perpetuate crises of human, animal and environmental health, and that their use is not only equitable for human communities that live with and rely upon animals but also for the animals that experience diseases associated with their living condition.

REFERENCES

Adam, K. E., Baillie, S., & Rushton, J. (2019). 'Clients. Outdoors. Animals.': Retaining vets in UK farm animal practice—Thematic analysis of free-text survey responses. *Vet Record, 184*(4), 121.

Anderson, A., & Hobson-West, P. (2022). "Refugees from practice?" Exploring why some vets move from the clinic to the laboratory. *Vet Record, 190*(1), e773.

Annand, E. J., Reid, P. A., Johnson, J., Gilbert, G. L., Taylor, M., Walsh, M., Ward, M. P., Wilson, A., & Degeling, C. (2020). Citizens' juries give verdict on whether private practice veterinarians should attend unvaccinated Hendra virus suspect horses. *Australian Veterinary Journal, 97*(7), 272–279.

Australian Veterinary Association. (2012). *Hendra Virus*. [Online]. https:// www.vetvoice.com.au/ec/diseases/hendra-virus/. Accessed 13 June 2023.

Australian Veterinary Association. (2016). *Hendra virus vaccine and its use by veterinary surgeons in Queensland.* Submission to the Queensland Parliament Agriculture and Environment Committee by the Australian Veterinary Association Ltd. Available at: https://documents.parliament.qld.gov.au/ committees/AEC/2016/rpt24-09-HendraVirusVacc/submissions/186.pdf. Accessed 13 June 2023.

Belshaw, Z., Robinson, N. J., Dean, R. S., & Brennan, M. L. (2018). Motivators and barriers for dog and cat owners and veterinary surgeons in the United

Kingdom to using preventative medicines. *Preventive Veterinary Medicine,* *154,* 95–101.

Bonnaud, L., & Fortané, N. (2020). Being a vet: The veterinary profession in social science research. *Review of Agricultural, Food and Environmental Studies, 102*(2), 125–149.

Bonnaud, L., & Fortané, N. (2021). 21st century vets: Professional dynamics in the era of One Health. *Review of Agricultural, Food and Environmental Studies, 102*(2), 121–124.

Bourgeois, L. F., Harell, A., & Stephenson, L. B. (2020). To Follow or not to follow: Social norms and civic duty during a pandemic. *Canadian Journal of Political Science, 53*(2), 273–278.

Chomel, B. B., Belotto, A., & Meslin, F.-X. (2007). Wildlife, exotic pets, and emerging zoonoses. *Emerging Infectious Diseases, 13,* 6–11.

Clarke, C., Knights, D., & Finch, G. (2016). Addressing disillusionment among young vets. *Vet Record, 179*(23), 603–604.

Daniel, A. (2023). *Hendra virus rarely spills from animals to us. Climate change makes it a bigger threat* [Online]. https://www.npr.org/sections/goatsa ndsoda/2022/11/16/1136850711/an-elegant-way-to-stop-deadly-hendra-virus-spillovers-from-bats-to-horses-to-us. Accessed 12 June 2023.

Davies, G. (2010). Captivating behaviour: Mouse models, experimental genetics and reductionist returns in the neurosciences. *The Sociological Review, 58*(1), 53–72.

Davies, G., Gorman, R., McGlacken, R., & Peres, S. (2022). The social aspects of genome editing: Publics as stakeholders, populations and participants in animal research. *Laboratory Animals, 56*(1), 88–96.

Degeling, C., & Kerridge, I. (2013). Hendra in the news: Public policy meets public morality in times of zoonotic uncertainty. *Social Science & Medicine, 82,* 156–163.

Ditlevsen, K., Glerup, C., Sandøe, P., & Lassen, J. (2020). Synthetic livestock vaccines as risky interference with nature? Lay and expert arguments and understandings of "naturalness." *Public Understanding of Science, 29*(3), 289–305.

Eschle, S., Hartmann, K., Rieger, A., Fischer, S., Kilma, A., & Bergmann, M. (2020). Canine vaccination in Germany: A survey of owner attitudes and compliance. *PLoS ONE, 15*(8), e0238371.

Evason, M., McGrath, M., & Stull, J. (2021). Companion animal preventive care at a veterinary teaching hospital—Knowledge, attitudes, and practices of clients. *The Canadian Veterinary Journal, 62*(5), 484–490.

Everitt, S., Pilnick, A., Waring, J., & Cobb, M. (2013). The structure of the small animal consultation. *Journal of Small Animal Practice, 54,* 453–458.

United Nations. (1968). *Feeding the expanding world population: International action to avert the impending protein crisis; report to the economic and social council.* United Nations.

Filipe, J. F. S., Lauzi, S., Pina, L., & Dall'Ara, P. (2021). A survey of Italian cat owners' attitudes towards cat vaccination through a web-based questionnaire. *BMC Veterinary Research, 17*, 267.

Galaz, V., Leach, M., Scoones, I., & Stein, C. (2015). *The political economy of One Health research and policy* (Working Paper Series: Political Economy of Knowledge and Polcy, 81). STEPS Centre.

Gardiner, A. (2014). The 'dangerous' Women of animal welfare: How British veterinary medicine went to the dogs. *Social History of Medicine, 27*(3), 466–487.

Gehrig, A.-C., Hartmann, K., Günther, F., Kilma, A., Habacher, G., & Bergmann, M. (2019). A survey of vaccine history in German cats and owners' attitudes to vaccination. *Journal of Feline Medicine and Surgery, 21*(2), 73–83.

Gibbs, E. P. J. (2014). The evolution of One Health: A decade of progress and challenges for the future. *Vet Record, 174*, 85–91.

Gilfoyle, D. (2006). Anthrax in South Africa: Economics, experiment and the mass vaccination of animals, c. 1910–1945. *Medical History, 50*, 465–490.

Gorman, R., & Davies, G. (2020). When 'cultures of care' meet: Entanglements and accountabilities at the intersection of animal research and patient involvement in the UK. *Social & Cultural Geography, 24*(1), 121–139.

Habacher, G., Gruffydd-Jones, T., & Murray, J. (2010). Use of a web-based questionnaire to explore cat owners' attitudes towards vaccination in cats. *Vet Record, 167*(4), 122–127.

Hagen, J. R., Weller, R., Mair, T. S., & Kinnison, T. (2020). Investigation of factors affecting recruitment and retention in the UK veterinary profession. *Vet Record, 187*(9), 354.

Hatch, P. H., Winefield, H. R., Christie, B. A., & Lievaart, J. J. (2011). Workplace stress, mental health, and burnout of veterinarians in Australia. *Australian Veterinary Journal, 89*(11), 460–468.

Craddock, S., & Hinchliffe, S. (2015). One world, one health? Social science engagements with the one health agenda. *Social Science & Medicine, 129*, 1–4.

Hinchliffe, S. (2015). More than one world, more than one health: Reconfiguring interspecies health. *Social Science and Medicine, 129*, 28–35.

Hobson-West, P. (2010). The role of 'public opinion' in the UK animal research debate. *Journal of Medical Ethics, 36*, 46–49.

McMichael, A. J., & Butler, C. D. (2007). Emerging health issues: The widening challenge for population health promotion. *Health Promotion International, 21*(S1), 15–24.

Mendez, D. H., Judd, J., & Speare, R. (2012). Unexpected result of Hendra virus outbreaks for veterinarians, Queensland, Australia. *Emerging Infectious Diseases, 18*, 83–85.

Middleton, D., Pallister, J., Klein, R., Feng, Y.-R., Haining, J., Arkinstall, R., Frazer, L., Huang, J.-A., Edwards, N., Wareing, M., Elhay, M., Hashmi, Z., Bingham, J., Yamada, M., Johnson, D., White, J., Foord, A., Heine, H. G., Marsh, G. A., … Wang, L.-F. (2014). Hendra virus vaccine, a one health approach to protecting horse, human, and environmental health. *Emerging Infectious Diseases, 20*(3), 372–379.

Monath, T. P. (2013). Vaccines against diseases transmitted from animals to humans: A one health paradigm. *Vaccine, 31*, 5321–5338.

Montoya, A. I. A., Hazel, S. J., Matthew, S. M., & McArthur, M. L. (2021). Why do veterinarians leave clinical practice? A qualitative study using thematic analysis. *Vet Record, 188*(1), 49–58.

Morris, P. (2012). *Blue Juice: Euthanasia in veterinary medicine*. Temple University Press.

Palmer, A., Message, R., & Greenhough, B. (2021). Edge cases in animal research law: Constituting the regulatory borderlands of the UK's animals (scientific procedures) act. *Studies in History and Philosophy of Science, 90*, 122–130.

Paolacci, G., & Chandler, J. (2014). Inside the Turk: Understanding mechanical Turk as a participant pool. *Current Directions in Psychological Science, 23*(3), 184–188.

PDSA. (2022). *PDSA animal wellbeing (PAW) report 2022* [Online]. https://www.pdsa.org.uk/media/12965/pdsa-paw-report-2022.pdf

Pedersen, H. (2014). Knowledge production in the "animal turn": Multiplying the image of thought, empathy, and justice. In E. A. Cederholm, A. Björck, K. Jennbert, & A.-S. Lönngren (Eds.), *Exploring the animal turn: Human-animal relations in science, society and culture* (pp. 13–18). Pufendorfinstitutet.

Pemberton, N., & Worboys, M. (2007). *Mad dogs and Englishmen: Rabies in Britain, 1830–2000*. Palgrave Macmillan.

Peres, S., & Roe, E. (2022). Laboratory animal strain mobilities: Handling with care for animal sentience and biosecurity. *History and Philosophy of the Life Sciences, 44*, 30.

Quick, T. (2023). *Flying monkeys and frogs in space: Towards a logistical history of laboratory animals*. Presentation at "Researching Animal Research", Wellcome Collection, 31st March 2023.

Ritvo, H. (2007). On the animal turn. *Daedalus, 136*(4), 118–122.

Robinson, N. J., Dean, R. S., Cobb, M., & Brennan, M. L. (2014). Consultation length in first opinion small animal practice. *Vet Record, 175*(19), 486–486.

Robinson, N. J., Brennan, M. L., & Cobb, M. (2015). Capturing the complexity of first opinion small animal consultations using direct observation. *Vet Record, 176*(2), 48.

Robinson, N, J., Belshaw, Z., Brennan, M. K. & Dean, R. S. (2019). Topics discussed, examinations performed and strategies implemented during canine and feline booster vaccination discussions. *Vet Record, 184*(8), 252–252.

Robinson, N., Dean, R., Brennan, M., & Belshaw, Z. (2022). The importance of preventative healthcare: What 10 years of research from the Centre for Evidence-based Veterinary Medicine reveals. *Companion Animal, 27*(3), 11–15.

Rusnock, A. (2009). Catching cowpox: The early spread of smallpox vaccination, 1798–1810. *Bulletin of the History of Medicine, 83*(1), 17–36.

Sánchez-Vizcaíno, F., Muniesa, A., Singleton, D. A., Jones, P. H., Noble, P. J., Gaskell, R. M., Dawson, S., & Radford, A. D. (2018). Use of vaccines and factors associated with their uptake variability in dogs, cats attending a large sentinel network veterinary practices across Great Britain. *Epidemiology & Infection, 146*, 895–903.

SAVSNET. (2016). *About SAVSNET* [Online]. https://www.liverpool.ac.uk/savsnet/about/. Accessed 12 June 2023.

Schemann, K., Annand, E. J., Reid, P. A., Lenz, M. F., Thomson, P. C., & Dhand, N. K. (2018). Investigation of the effect of Equivac® HeV Hendra virus vaccination on Thoroughbred racing performance. *Australian Veterinary Journal, 96*(4), 132–141.

Schwedinger, E., Kuhne, F., & Moritz, A. (2021). What influence do vets have on vaccination decision of dog owners? Results of an online survey. *Vet Record,* e297.

Shaw, J. R., Adams, C. L., Bonnett, B. N., Larson, S., & Roter, D. L. (2008). Veterinarian-client-patient communication during wellness appointments versus appointments related to a health problem in companion animal practice. *Journal of the American Veterinary Medicine Association, 233*(10), 1576–1586.

Swabe, J. (1999). *Animals, disease and human society: Human-animal relations and the rise of veterinary medicine.* Routledge.

Tan, R. H. H., Hodge, A., Klein, R., Edwards, N., Huang, J. A., Middleton, D., & Watts, S. P. (2018). Virus-neutralising antibody responses in horses following vaccination with Euivac® HeV: A field study. *Australian Veterinary Journal, 96*(5), 161–166.

Vanderslott, S., Palmer, A., Thomas, T., Greenhough, B., Stuart, A., Henry, J. A., English, M., Naude, R. D. W., Patrick-Smith, M., Douglas, N., Moore, M., Hodgson, S. H., Emary, K. R.W, & Pollard, A. J. (2021). Co-producing human and animal experimental subjects: Exploring the views of UK COVID-19 vaccine trial participants on animal testing. *Science, Technology, & Human Values*, in press.

Volk, J. O., Felsted, K. E., Thomas, J. G., & Siren, C. W. (2011). Executive summary of the Bayer veterinary care usage study. *Journal of American Veterinary Medicine Association, 238*(10), 12751282.

World Organisation for Animal Health. (2011). *No more deaths from rinderpest* [Online]. https://www.woah.org/en/no-more-deaths-from-rinderpest/. Accessed 12 June 2023.

Wolfe, C. (2011). Moving forward, kicking back: The animal turn. *Postmedieval: A Journal of Medieval Cultural Studies, 2*, 1–12.

Woods, A., & Bresalier, M. (2014). One health, many histories. *Vet Record, 174*(26), 650–654.

Woods, A. (2007). The farm as clinic: Veterinary expertise and the transformation of dairy farming, 1930–1950. *Studies in the History and Philosophy of Biology and Biomedical Science, 38*, 462–487.

Woods, A. (2017). From one medicine to two: The evolving relationship between human and veterinary medicine in England, 1791–1835. *Bulletin of the History of Medicine, 91*, 494–523.

Woods, A. T., Velasco, C., Levitan, C. A., Wan, X., & Spence, C. (2015). Conducting perception research over the internet: A tutorial review. *PeerJ, 3*, e1058.

Woods, A., Bresalier, M., Cassidy, A., & Dentinger, R. M. (2018). *Animals and the shaping of modern medicine: One health and its histories*. Springer Nature.

Yuen, K. Y., Fraser, N. S., Henning, J., Halpin, K., Gibson, J. S., Betzien, L., & Stewart, A. J. (2021). Hendra virus: Epidemiology dynamics in relation to climate change, diagnostic tests and control measures. *One Health, 12*, 100207.

CHAPTER 7

Conclusion

Abstract This chapter draws our arguments together to provide an overarching picture of how societies engineer high levels of vaccine coverage, as well as the central challenges or limitations that threaten high levels of uptake. Furthermore, we examine the benefits of the conceptual approach that we have adopted in this book and offer a clear example of the significance that this broader social and political analysis of vaccines holds for continued analysis of the specific problem of vaccine hesitancy. This chapter therefore offers an analysis of the interconnections between critical public views commonly examined by social scientists, and the social and political components of the broader (and initially seemingly unconnected) workings of the immunisation social order and the actors that comprise it which we have examined in Vaccines in Society.

Keywords Immunisation Social Order · Pharmaceutical Controversy · Vaccine Hesitancy · Distrust · Science Communication

7.1   The Nature, Functioning and Limits of the Immunisation Social Order

Vaccines are thoroughly social and political. In this book—looking beyond only or primarily the social and political basis of hesitant or critical public and parental understandings—we have revealed the myriad ways in which this is so. We have focused on several dimensions from across what Kirkland (2016) calls the 'immunisation social order'. As we have discussed, this concept involves or reveals a broad yet fragile web of institutional, scientific, legal—and importantly—social and political practices, associated actors and relationships that produce and protect high levels of vaccination coverage. The concept is a highly valuable one. As this book demonstrates, the utility of the concept of the immunisation social order for social scientists is to be found particularly in the analytical attention it directs towards the range of sociological and political factors underpinning how high levels of vaccination coverage are achieved and maintained, as well as the challenges, restrictions and limitations that may prevent or threaten high levels of vaccination coverage—beyond only vaccine hesitancy—in specific national contexts but also internationally.

The book began with a historical overview of the social and political dimensions of vaccine science and the associated growth of the immunisation social order as well as emerging challenges and tensions within it. For example, we were able to show that the development of the smallpox vaccine and thus the beginnings of the immunisation social order—rather than emerging from individual scientific genius as the story of Edward Jenner suggests—reflected the socially situated nature of knowledge production. More broadly, the chapter highlighted how the political and economic order has shaped vaccine science with new vaccines, or the need for them, also in turn reshaping societies. Furthermore, the chapter emphasised the importance of co-operation (for example, co-operation across the Cold War ideological divide led to the eradication of smallpox). We additionally discussed challenges and tensions within the emerging immunisation social order. As neoliberalism spread globally, we have argued that there was a growing divergence between public health need and private corporate interests in the development of vaccines and threats to the supply of vaccines poised by litigation when a small number of individuals are harmed by vaccination. New legislation to protect the supply and the emergence of public–private partnerships to incentivise vaccine development partially resolved these problems and reshaped vaccine development and society in the process.

We then examined the presence of social values and the political nature of vaccines in the context of the modern-day development and regulation of vaccines. In one example, we discussed how gender norms and heteronormativity were embedded in how the first HPV vaccine was developed and targeted which restricted optimal levels of vaccine coverage and thus the optimal functioning of the immunisation social order. In another example, we demonstrated the centrality of social values in regulatory decision-making and the subsequent withdrawal of the first rotavirus vaccine in the USA despite health authorities initially providing an ostensibly epidemiological justification. This example highlighted how social values and sociocultural context influence which vaccines are used and the associated level of acceptable risk as evaluated by regulators—and, as such, the composition, nature and functioning of the immunisation social order. Finally, through a focus on the development of COVID-19 vaccines, we analysed not only the bespoke approach adopted by key actors in the development and regulation of COVID-19 vaccines, but also how the interests of powerful groups were reflected in the approaches to development and regulation and thus the composition and functioning of the immunisation social order during the COVID-19 pandemic.

Furthermore, we have examined the role played by various forms of media within the immunisation social order. We analysed the role played by journalists in the co-production of representations and understandings of vaccines. Through the concept of biomediatisation we began to analyse the entanglements between biomedicine and media/journalism and the influence of each sector/profession on the other. Drawing on evidence relating to swine flu vaccination, we examined how journalistic practices influence how vaccines are represented, understood, and their societal perceptions co-produced. Though journalistic practices may conceivably challenge or criticise the functioning of the immunisation social order, the evidence also suggests that journalists use their social position to constrain the spread of illegitimate vaccine opinion and thus help to maintain and preserve high levels of vaccination coverage. The fluid landscape of social media was finally surveyed as an area ripe with tools for proponents and opponents of the immunisation social order, and an uncertain methodological and interventional future.

The layered complexity of social and economic inequalities associated with vaccine access and uptake were assessed in chapter five. We argued that the inequalities surrounding vaccines operated in multiple directions with social justice impacts arising where the immunisation social order demonstrates penetration and effectiveness, but unequal economic and social conditions acting to restrict this same penetration and effectiveness. We contended that in the current makeup of the immunisation social order, vaccine inequalities present something of an ouroboros: while economic incentives are required to drive some areas of innovation and scaling in the pharmaceutical industry required to fulfil the aims of the immunisation social order, these same incentives are absent in economically deprived areas of the world that may benefit the most from access to vaccines.

Finally, we explored the historic and current relationships between non-human animals and the technology of vaccination. From early challenges arising from the geographic spread of cowpox through to the contemporary enmeshment of social attitudes around animal research and the evaluation of risk in the immunisation social order, we illustrated some of the ways that the immunisation social order has absorbed and enacts aspects of the veterinary-driven philosophy of One Health. As with previous chapters, we highlighted some of the indirect impacts of the functioning of the immunisation social order on issues around animal preservation.

7.2   The Utility of a Broader Sociological Understanding of Vaccines

In this final section of the book, we wish to provide a clear example of the significance that a broader social and political analysis of vaccines holds for continued analysis of the specific problem of vaccine hesitancy. In other words, this section offers an analysis of the interconnections between critical public views and the social and political components of the broader (and initially seemingly unconnected) workings of the immunisation social order and the actors that comprise it drawing particularly on arguments made by Goldenberg (2021).

Despite the lengthy time frame and the robust regulatory processes that are associated with vaccine development and testing, the most cited reason for vaccine hesitancy in the general population is safety concern (Yaqub et al., 2014). Research similarly shows us that another prominent concern held by the vaccine hesitant is distrust in the government/

health authorities and the pharmaceutical industry (ibid.; Reich, 2016).[1] In this sense, evidence reveals that the most important reasons why some people are hesitant or reject vaccination relate to the processes and actors that develop and ensure the efficacy and safety of vaccines within the immunisation social order.

Why do vaccine-critical people distrust the pharmaceutical industry? In large part, this is because of the commercialisation of science and medical research—and associated concerns about conflicts of interest—that has gradually intensified since the second half of the twentieth century (Larson, 2018). In other words, even though the pharmaceutical industry has generated many life-improving and lifesaving products, it is also focused on generating profit, and this provokes public concern about their motives—including relating to the production of vaccines.

Many within medicine and the pharmaceutical sector dismiss valid concerns relating to commercialised medical science (Goldenberg, 2021). In relation to vaccines, actors within the pharmaceutical industry often contend that the vaccine market is not especially profitable, particularly compared to 'blockbuster' drugs, and that pharmaceutical companies have left or have considered leaving the market many times in the past. Concern about conflicts of interest, unethical practices (such as hiding damaging data), pharmaceutical harm (for example, the opioid crisis) and product withdrawals are minimised or dismissed, and instead these actors point to the life-improving and lifesaving nature of some of their products which does not help assuage concern (ibid.).

It is true that at times the discourse surrounding pharmaceutical controversies and conflicts of interest can stray into the realm of conspiracy theory. But it is also true that a considerable body of research reveals the existence of very real problems within the pharmaceuticals sector. A range of social analyses have revealed the problematic influences and practices of the pharmaceutical industry throughout the processes of research, regulation, guideline development and decision-making about pharmaceutical products (see Light et al., 2013; Rodwin, 2013). Indeed, over three decades sociologist John Abraham (1995, 2002, 2008, 2010) has carefully analysed what he calls corporate bias in the development and regulation of pharmaceutical products (or, in other words the privileged

[1] Lack of trust in the pharmaceutical industry and health authorities is similarly associated with vaccine hesitancy among medical professionals (Manca, 2018; Verger et al., 2022).

strategic—and secretive—involvement of the pharmaceutical industry in government regulatory policy and outcomes). Broadly speaking, his body of work—comprising many peer-reviewed journal papers and a range of books—argues that social forces, particularly relating to the interests of the pharmaceutical industry, may exaggerate or distort the perceived need for, utility of or safety of pharmaceutical products and result in the inefficient use of healthcare funding/resources (see Douglass, 2023 for an overview).

Following Goldenberg (2021), the point here is not to argue that these issues *necessarily* impact vaccines in development or use today in global vaccination programmes/schedules. Rather, it is to argue that the public are aware of the very real range of pharmaceutical controversies, conflicts of interest, scandals and inquiries into injury and death within the sector the perception of which are co-produced by journalists who report on this topic. This influences how the public understand vaccines and can lead to distrust in the pharmaceutical industry and government regulators. Building trust in vaccines and the actors that develop and regulate them also relates to how science is communicated to the public by the institutions of the immunisation social order. As has long been shown in science and technology studies, science, including pharmaceutical science, involves uncertainty (Caudill, 2023). However, during the COVID-19 pandemic in Britain, for example, science was largely presented as certain even as policies informed by that same science widely fluctuated under the banner of 'following the science'. The pandemic was also marked by some level of tendency to dismiss or demonise the views of people who hold a non-consensus science worldview—an approach that was unlikely to be effective in persuading people to accept COVID-19 vaccination. Framing someone as 'unintelligent' or 'misinformed' for holding vaccine-critical views is likely only to prompt an angry reaction, and is unlikely to result in a radical change of their perspective. Instead, Caudill (2023) argues that effective science communication should involve listening and attempts to understand by the institutions of the immunisation social order why some people hold a non-consensus science worldview. He argues it should also involve humility and modesty on the part of scientists reflecting the uncertainties inherent in science.

To build impactful science communication strategies, we need to understand and sufficiently appreciate the importance of social and political forces. Central to this endeavour must be recognition that the values, experiences, interests and social positions held across society influence how scientific knowledge—including information about vaccine safety and regulatory processes—is received, understood and acted on. Overall, a sociological approach like the one we have adopted in this book that reveals the influence of social and political forces on the very nature of vaccines, on how we come to know them as well as the full range of their social impacts can help in turn to cast further light on the underpinnings and dynamics of societal caution around vaccines and the urgings of the collective components of the immunisation social order.

REFERENCES

Abraham, J. (1995). *Science, politics and the pharmaceutical industry*. UCL Press.
Abraham, J. (2002). Drug safety and the safety of patients: The challenge to medicine and health from permissive expert risk assessments of triazolam (Halcion). *Health, Risk and Society, 4*(1), 19–29. https://doi.org/10.1080/13698570210292
Abraham, J. (2008). Sociology of pharmaceuticals development and regulation: A realist empirical research programme. *Sociology of Health & Illness, 30*(6), 869–885. https://doi.org/10.1111/j.1467-9566.2008.01101.x
Abraham, J. (2010). Pharmaceuticalization of society in context: Theoretical, empirical and health dimensions. *Sociology, 44*(4), 603–622. https://doi.org/10.1177/0038038510369368
Caudill, D. S. (2023). *Expertise in crisis: The ideological contours of public scientific controversies*. Policy Press.
Douglass, T. (2023). Conceptual tools for the analysis of bioeconomic fairness and efficiency. *Asian Biotechnology and Development Review, 25*(1&2), 23–35. https://www.ris.org.in/sites/default/files/2023-08/ABDR-March-July-2023.pdf
Goldenberg, M. J. (2021). *Vaccine hesitancy: Public trust, expertise, and the war on science*. University of Pittsburgh Press.
Kirkland, A. (2016). *Vaccine court: The law and politics of injury*. NYU Press.
Larson, H. J. (2018). Politics and public trust shape vaccine risk perceptions. *Nature Human Behaviour, 2*(5), 316–316. https://doi.org/10.1038/s41562-018-0331-6
Light, D. W., Lexchin, J., & Darrow, J. J. (2013). Institutional corruption of pharmaceuticals and the myth of safe and effective drugs. *Journal of Law, Medicine & Ethics, 41*(3), 590–600. https://doi.org/10.1111/jlme.12068
Manca, T. (2018). "One of the greatest medical success stories": Physicians and nurses' small stories about vaccine knowledge and anxieties. *Social Science & Medicine, 196*, 182–189.
Reich, J. A. (2016). *Calling the shots*. New York University Press.

Rodwin, M. A. (2013). Institutional corruption and the pharmaceutical policy. *Journal of Law, Medicine & Ethics, 41*(3), 544–552.

Verger, P., Botelho-Nevers, E., Garrison, A., Gagnon, D., Gagneur, A., Gagneux-Brunon, A., & Dubé, E. (2022). Vaccine hesitancy in health-care providers in Western countries: A narrative review. *Expert Review of Vaccines, 21*(7), 909–927.

Yaqub, O., Castle-Clarke, S., Sevdalis, N., & Chataway, J. (2014). Attitudes to vaccination: A critical review. *Social Science & Medicine, 112*, 1–11. https://doi.org/10.1016/j.socscimed.2014.04.018

INDEX

A
Animal-related challenges in the
   distribution of vaccines, 86
Animals, 84–89, 92–101
   agency, 86
   public opinion, 93, 94, 100
   social scientific attention, 84

B
BCG vaccine, 17
Biocommunicability, 51
Biomediatisation, 48, 49, 58
Burden of disease, 66

C
Centre for Disease Control (CDC),
   39–41
Cold War divide, 17
Commercialised medical science, 111
Conflicts of interest, 111, 112
Co-production, 49, 51, 52, 58
Corporate bias, 111
COVAX, 70

COVID-19 pandemic, 2, 6, 7
COVID-19 vaccine, 2, 3, 7, 41–44,
   68–71, 74
   manufacturing capacity, 69
   national interest, 70
   nationalism, 70
COVID-19 vaccine development, 34,
   42
   regulation, 42
Cowpox, 13, 14
Cultural representations of vaccines,
   58
Cutter Incident, 19

D
Development and regulation of
   vaccines, 44
Diphtheria-tetanus-pertussis (DTP)
   combination vaccine, 20

E
Ebola Virus Disease, 88
Eradication of smallpox, 18